God's Healing Herbs

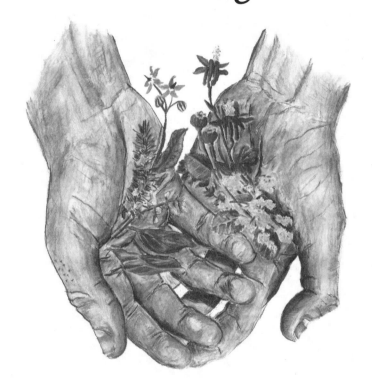

God's Healing Herbs

by

DENNIS ELLINGSON

Illustrations by Matthew Kondratieff

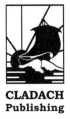

CLADACH
Publishing

DISCLAIMER:
Information in this book is not intended to be taken as a replacement for medical
advice. Any person with a condition requiring medical attention should consult a
qualified health practitioner or therapist.

Library of Congress Control Number: 2006920012

ISBN-13: 978-0-975961-93-3
ISBN-10: 0-975961-934

Printed in the U.S.A.

Contents

Dedicated to the Lord God, who was
"walking in the garden in the cool of the day" (Gen. 3:8).

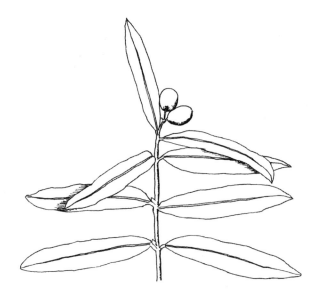

Introduction

The purpose of this book is threefold. First, to introduce you to the family of herbs, as I have been discovering them, for their healing aspects as well as their spiritual attributes. Second, to introduce you to another aspect of God as the One who desires to provide for and sustain your good health through what He has created for you. Third, to help you discover "living parables"—comparisons of the natural world with God's spiritual world.

First let me state that I am not in any way a medical authority. This book is for your reference and entertainment only. It is not a medical manual. I am simply a Christian pastor and writer who has sought, like you, to find natural ways to improve and maintain health. Because of the powerful nature of some herbs discussed here, do consult your physician before using them. I am in no way giving medical advice. My research comes from many sources.

As a man in middle life, I am taking nutrition much more seriously than ever before; but perhaps not for the reason you might think. I am now concerned with the quality of the life I live, but less about how long I will live. The length of our lives is God's affair. But the quality of our lives is much more up to us.

Eating and living healthily is more desirous as I watch myself age. I don't mind the aging process—there is nothing I can do about the advance of years—but I do want to age well. If quality foods spiced with herbs will improve my health, stamina, and vitality; keep me more fit for life and service; then my life and service will be more enjoyable.

When the first edition of *God's Healing Herbs* came out I had a few hopes for it. One, that it would honor God, the Creator, who has provided these herbs for us. Two, that people would learn to increase their knowledge about the beneficial power of herbs for spirit, mind, and body. And third, that this book would become a standard perennial guide added to from time to time.

Because of the readers' appreciation of this book, my first and second hopes continue to be realized, and now with this new updated and expanded version, so has my third hope.

I am also concerned because the field of herbal study has long been one that has leaned toward the occult, witchcraft, and other earth-bound religions. To give an example: In searching for sources for my research, the name Gaia often appears. It could be included in the name of an herb grower or company, or a product name. It is important to understand that the name Gaia is rooted in the occult. Gaia is the supposed mother earth god. For the occultist this earthly creation that the one true God has provided for us as a place to live and take care of, has become god itself. The Bible foretold of this: "They exchange the truth of God for a lie, and worshipped and served created things rather than the Creator—who is forever praised. Amen" (Rom. 1:25).

I believe that through this book you will be drawn to a deeper understanding of God as Creator.

In this book I list descriptions of numerous herbs. Many of these are mentioned in the Bible or have a spiritual link. For the most part, I have included herbs that are my favorites and that have shown a "track record" in their benefits. Also mentioned are fruits, vegetables, and flowers that you may not have considered as herbs, but they are included here because of their healing qualities.

I will give you advice for planting and growing herbs, sources of where to buy them, recipes for cooking with them, and more. This resource is not meant to be all-inclusive. With thousands of plant species growing on this great earth, the list could be almost endless.

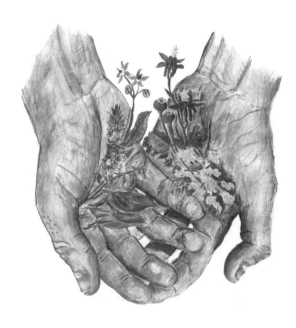

The Herbs A to Z
~ Contents ~

The Herbs A to Z

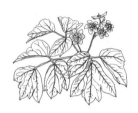 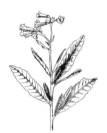

KEY TO HERBAL ICONS

⚙ Description

⚙ Growing Tips

⚙ Medicinal Parts

⚙ Internal Uses

⚙ External Uses

⚙ Culinary Uses

☞ How to Prepare

📔 Biblical References

❗ Cautionary Concerns

Note: If one of these symbols does not occur under a particular herb, then there are no specific recommendations noted for that herb.

Alfalfa

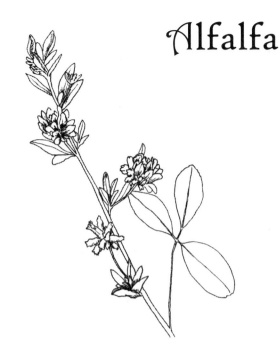

Journeying out and about in the rural farmland of central and eastern Oregon during haying season, the sweet, healthy scent of fresh-cut alfalfa speaks of good things to come.

⊞ A legume, alfalfa is grown as an annual or perennial. The plant grows 12 to 18 inches high. Look for blue to purple flowers in August, then seed pods. Rich in nutrients. High in chlorophyll, this herb is a natural deodorizer and detoxifier. A good source of calcium, magnesium, potassium. Rich in vitamins A and K.

✿ Grow inside in a sprouting jar. A tablespoon of seeds in a quart jar produces plenty of sprouts in four days. To grow the plants, you need well-drained, loamy soil. And a drier climate is best. Sow seed ¼ inch deep and water regularly until established, then fairly drought tolerant. Most farmers plant alfalfa in the fall for full development in the spring. Also grown because it benefits the soil.

❀ Flowers, leaves, petals, and sprouted seeds.

✋ A cancer fighter rich in beta-carotene. Helpful for the heart, it may lower high blood pressure. A great laxative and a digestive aid that may help with gastritis, intestinal ulcers and hemorrhoids. Good for urinary tract and bladder infections and acts as a natural diuretic. A centuries-old remedy for the symptoms of arthritis and rheumatism. There are indications that it can help with liver disorders, eczema, asthma, anemia, and many other conditions, from bleeding gums to athlete's foot. It's also suggested that women who have a likelihood for miscarriage should utilize alfalfa. Why are we just letting the cattle of the field take advantage of all this goodness?

🍽 Try a little in a salad, purchase sprouts at the store or grow your own.

☞ Best used in fresh form. Many people use alfalfa as tea. You may look for a high quality product in capsule or liquid form at your local health store.

📖 The name seems to come from the Muslims. *AL* for Allah and *FALF* for "Father of all Foods." However, I like Psalm 104:14-24: "He [God] makes grass grow for the cattle, and plants for man to cultivate—bringing forth food from the earth.... How many are your works, O Lord! In wisdom you made them all."

❗ This is a powerful herb, so a little goes a long way. There is concern that if you have an autoimmune disease, such as lupus, alfalfa in more than moderate amounts could aggravate the condition. Check with your doctor before using.

Almond

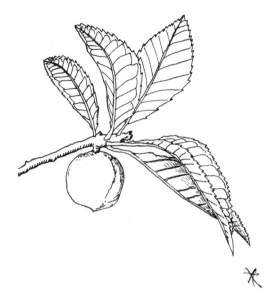

⊞ Cultivated in warmer areas of the West. The tree grows to 20 feet, with serrated leaves, thorny branches, and large white flowers.

☼ Best grown in areas where the last frost comes before April.

🌹 Nut or kernel

🍵 Studies suggest that almond oil may help prevent heart disease and lower serum cholesterol levels. Eat the nut whole or ground; or extract the essential oil. Nuts are enjoying a resurgence in popularity for their health benefits, and almond is no exception. Oil from the bitter almond is a good remedy for coughs.

✳ Facial scrub. The emollient properties can remove excess oil and dirt from skin, as well as moisturize and soften.

🍽 I like almond butter as an alternative to peanut butter. Find in health food sections or grind your own. Provides energy for high-exertion, such as hiking.

☞ Consume the nut whole, ground, or pressed (oil extract).

📖 Consider Jeremiah 1:11-12. "The word of the Lord came to me: 'What do you see, Jeremiah?' 'I see the branch of an almond tree,' I replied. The Lord said to me, 'You have seen correctly, for I am watching to see that my word is fulfilled.'" In the Bible lands, the almond is one of the first blooms of the year, appearing as early as January or February, signifying that even in the depths of winter, there is hope of spring. God uses this to illustrate that he will fulfill his ultimate plan.

As winter wears on, I can hardly wait for spring. Where I live, we sometimes get a false spring early in the new year, causing hope that winter will be short; but winter always comes back. Likewise, the long winter of the fallen world we live in seems long, but it will not always last. The promise of a new earth, new heaven, and new Jerusalem will come to pass. Just as the almond tree will bloom, so will God's ultimate plan. Look up then, your redemption and your Lord draw near!

Aaron, Moses' brother, carried a rod of almond wood, and the Lord made it blossom and bear fruit. He did this as a sign of promise, so that the Hebrews would stop grumbling and believe that God would deliver them.

Aloe Vera

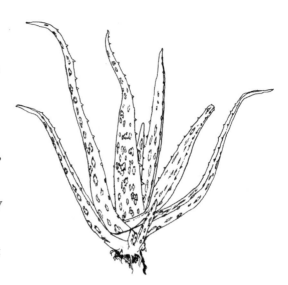

⊞ A wonderful plant! A species of the day lily, aloe vera grows long, tubular leaves filled with clear sap.

☼ Grows well indoors (and outdoors in some areas). Very prolific—continually spawns off new plants. In a short time, from a group of shoots, you can have numerous plants. It needs little water, prefers sandy soil, and doesn't need a lot of care. Cutting a branch off for use has little negative effect upon the plant.

🌷 Use the leaves.

☞ Some people utilize aloe vera for internal purposes, such as digestive problems and arthritis. Before doing this, consult your pharmacist or health care professional as to the best and safest method. Professionally-processed juice and capsules are the safer way to go.

🏘 Aloe Vera's healing properties soothe skin scrapes, irritations, and sunburns. Because I like to spend time outdoors, I am frequently treating sunburn. You can use the natural gel or emollient from the cut leaves; or buy a 100% aloe ointment. Keep it in the refrigerator and get a double cooling effect. It is also said to be good for chickenpox and acne. Ladies like to use it after shaving their legs. The substance is used in radiation burns; and it seems to have a positive effect in counteracting scarring. (Aloe has astringent, or drying qualities, so does not act as a moisturizer unless it is combined with a moisturizing substance.)

☞ Cut a leaf from the plant, squeeze out the sap and spread liberally on affected skin area.

📖 According to W. E. Shewell-Cooper, it is the perfume qualities of the aloe that are mentioned in Numbers, Psalms, Proverbs, Song of Solomon, and John.

Aloe was probably one of the embalming spices Nicodemus and Joseph of Arimathea used for the crucified body of Jesus.

The aloes mentioned in the Bible are perfumes that likely came from a tree in India known as "Eaglewood." The aloe mentioned in John 19:39 is from the lily family, the same one we use for topical medicinal purposes.

❢ If using externally, don't combine or use along with licorice. Check with your doctor first if you are on prescribed steroid use or heart medicines.

Angelica

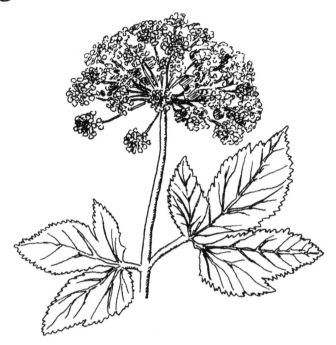

▣ The angelica plant is also known as "master-wort" because of its many uses. Blossoms of greenish-white flowers grow in compound umbels that exude a honey-like aroma. The plant bears an oblong fruit with two seeds in each pod.

☼ A perennial that grows easily, but may reach 8 feet tall and self-sows easily. Prefers a rich, damp soil, but tolerates many conditions.

❀ Rootstock and seeds.

⬗ Said to have a warming effect upon the body and to improve circulation. May be helpful during painful menstrual cycles. Said to be helpful for treating colds, coughs, tensions, headache, flu, insomnia, and for easier breathing.

👬 Rub on skin for gout and rheumatic conditions; or to get rid of skin lice. For sore muscles, try angelica in your bath. Add to potpourri.

🍽 Leaves can be used in salads, soups, and stews; or use in fruit drinks and iced teas. Note a somewhat sweet taste.

☞ Cut and dry the rootstock in its second year. Boil seeds for a tea infusion, or grind them to a powder.

📖 None noted. The name angelica comes from a French Catholic legend that says the angel Raphael revealed the secrets of this herb to a monk for use during a plague epidemic.

❗ Avoid use if pregnant, diabetic, or if you are taking blood-thinning medications.

Anise

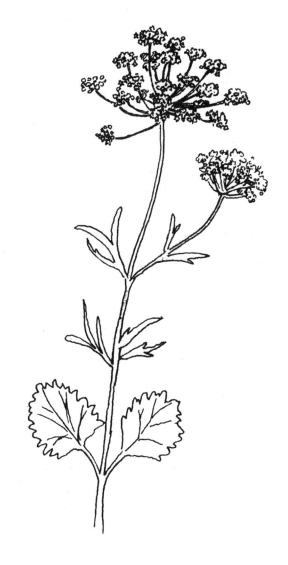

▣ An annual that grows to a height of 18 inches. Anise has compound umbel flowers with a fragrant aroma. An easy plant to grow in your garden.

☼ Likes sun, and doesn't need a lot of water.

🌿 The seeds.

🍵 Brewed and consumed as a tea, anise is said to help with digestion problems, gas, nausea, and cramps. It is also used during colds to help relieve congestion. For your baby, you might find it will help with colic; but check with your physician first. For nursing mothers, recent scientific studies show that it may improve milk production.

🍽 The leaves, stalks, and seeds can be utilized in a number of ways to spice up a variety of dishes. I use the oil to attract trout when I am fishing and it seems to work!

☞ Crush the dried seeds gently to release the volatile oils, then steep 1 teaspoon crushed seeds in 1 cup boiling water. Drink as a tea.

📖 Recorded in Matthew 23:23 as one of the herbs used for tithing. From anise we get the flavor of licorice.

Apple

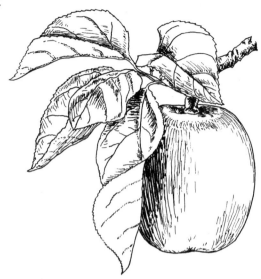

⚜ Fruit from the common apple tree of which there are many varieties.

🌻 The whole fruit

🗝 "An Apple a day keeps the doctor away." The old adage could very well be true. If William Tell lived today and was concerned about his health, though, he wouldn't shoot the apple off his son's head. He'd eat it. Apples are a great tonic for the stomach. They help diarrhea or constipation. I've found that an apple is a great way to curb a touch of indigestion or upset stomach without resorting to antacid medicine. Apples are high in fiber, yet gentle on your system; they lower cholesterol, normalize blood sugar, and may be helpful for rheumatism.

🍽 Many. When recipes call for sugar, try substituting apple juice or applesauce. You will get the sweetness you want in a more healthful way.

📖 There is no evidence that it was an apple with which the serpent enticed Eve. We don't know what the fruit was, but it's no longer present on this earth. Two trees mentioned in the Garden of Eden story are no longer found on earth: the Tree of Life and the Tree of the Knowledge of Good and Evil. These trees had some sort of fruit on them. Adam and Eve were commanded not to eat from the Tree of the Knowledge of Good and Evil. Everything else was acceptable. When humankind, through Adam and Eve, fell into sin, these trees were removed.

I believe there is a relationship between this tree and the cross of Christ. If Adam and Eve (and we are no different than they) had been obedient, then the Son would not have had to die for us on another tree.

Psalm 1:3 tells us to be like a tree planted near streams of water, flourishing and prospering in a never-ending flow of living water. Let apples remind you of God's love and care. "In a desert land he found him, in a barren and howling waste. He shielded him and cared for him; he guarded him as the apple of his eye" (Deut. 32:10).

Artichoke

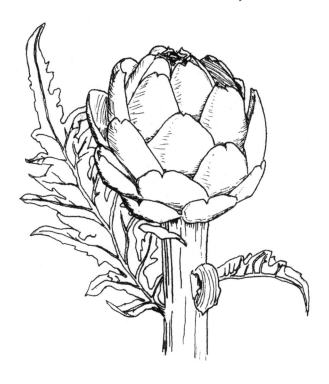

🏵 A perennial plant from the Mediterranean. Used worldwide as a unique and fun food source. Plant grows a long tuber root, a stem reaching to 5 feet high with spiny leaves. The plant blossoms blue flowers that are a part of the flower head which is what most of us consume.

☼ In harsh climates, artichoke is grown as an annual. Optimum conditions seem to be like what you would find on the California coast, with cool summers. Start plant in early spring or fall, depending upon climate, in raised beds and take measures to control slugs, snails, and aphids all of which love the plant.

🌿 Flower or fruit, leaves and root.

🗹 From the leaves, extracts are said to help in preventing hardening of the arteries and to treat dyspepsia, liver function, anemia, and jaundice. It may be another fine herb you can enjoy that has diuretic properties, so it also may help lower high blood pressure and cholesterol.

🍽 Enjoy it steamed in a little water, olive oil, and red wine vinegar for ½ hour to 45 minutes, or until tender.

❗ None noted, but artichoke is high in fiber so if you are not used to a high fiber diet, start with moderation.

Asparagus

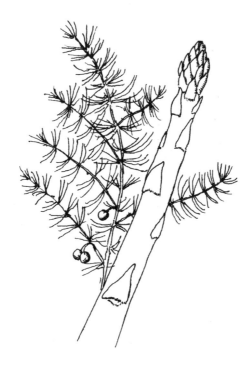

⊞ A perennial garden plant that grows wild in North America. My grandmother and I used to pick it out of irrigation ditches. The root of the plant sends up long shoots which are harvested for use. Asparagus plants also grow delicate, fern-like leaves that make nice ornamentals.

☼ Asparagus grows in loose, dryer soil, and takes 2 years to produce edible fruit, but it may give you 10 to 12 years of crops.

⚘ Young shoots or spears.

⎇ Asparagus is helpful to the kidneys and seems to have a cleansing effect upon them and the urinary tract. You may notice a stronger urine smell after eating them. Because the plant is high in fiber, it will certainly help regulate and speed up the digestion process. The plant contains folic acid which is good for red blood cell development. It may even help in easing a toothache and an aching back! And it is considered an aphrodisiac.

🍽 Good in salads, though I don't eat it raw. High in vitamins A and C.

☞ I cook asparagus in the same manner I cook artichoke.

❗ Since it does act on the kidneys, if you are already having kidney problems, you will want to avoid eating asparagus or check with your doctor first.

Balm

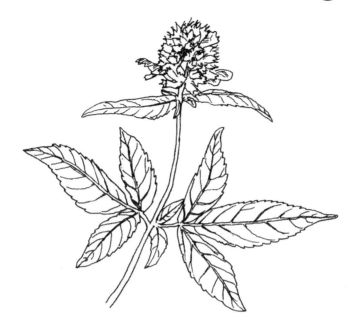

❀ This is a perennial plant, sometimes grown as an annual, with numerous varieties. My favorites are lemon balm and bee balm. Related to the mint family.

☼ Grows easily, and will overrun a garden; better to keep these plants in a pot. It will "die" in winter; but new branches and leaves will come up in the spring.

🌿 The leaves.

📯 A calmative and digestive aid that also helps with insomnia, gas, and even asthma. Balms are used for herbal teas. Lemon balm gives your tea a lemon twist. Indians introduced bee balm to the Pilgrims. It was used as an alternative to Earl Grey tea during the American Revolutionary War. Remember from your history books about the "Tea Party" in Boston Harbor, when the tea was dumped into the sea as a tax protest?

👪 Try it in a bath; tuck it in a pillow. A poultice of balm may relieve sores, rashes, and insect bites.

🍽 Try fresh, tender leaves in a salad.

☞ Use fresh or dried leaves in boiling water for a tea.

📖 A "Balm in Gilead" is mentioned in Jeremiah 8:22. This is a different kind of balm—the resin from a tree, rather than the leafy bushes mentioned above. The word "balm" suggests comfort to the mind and body. In the Bible, references to balm are always parabolic in that it is our Lord who gives us comfort and rest for our souls. Balm is a reminder to us of the comfort we can enjoy in having salvation, grace, ever-present relationship, presence, power, and healing in our lives through Jesus Christ.

Barley

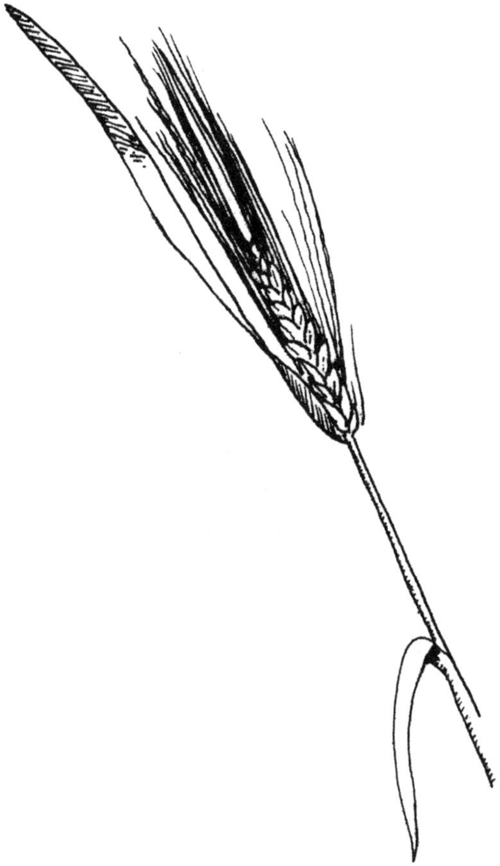

An annual plant used for millenniums around the world as a food source. Barley grows to 3 feet tall, with bristle-like flowers that eventually develop into the grain and seed.

An agricultural crop that adapts to many climates, ripens quickly, and is heat-resistant. You could try growing some in a small area as an ornamental.

The grain.

While considered the "poor man's grain," barley is full of nutrients, minerals, vitamins, and antioxidants. Hulled pearl barley seems to make eating easier for those with throat or stomach problems. Barley may also have a soothing effect upon the stomach and the intestines, and it is an old-time recommendation as a food to serve a person with a fever.

Cooked barley has been used as an external application for skin sores, such as boils.

Many. For instance, if you just have to have your beef, then try a beef-and-barley soup, and the barley will aid in a quicker digestion.

Boil 2 ounces of washed barley in 4 pints of water for internal or external use.

A common food of the people, barley is mentioned numerous times. In Exodus 9:31, barley was destroyed in the plague of hail. In Numbers 5:15, it was used as an offering. In I Kings 4:28 barley was used as fodder for animals.

Gideon had a strange dream where a huge loaf of barley bread rolled into the enemy's tent and destroyed it (Judges 7:13). This dream prophesied that Israel, though small and inferior like barley, would with God's help defeat the Midians, considered to be superior, as were wheat and other grains.

My favorite barley story is Jesus' feeding of the multitudes. With the kind gift of a poor boy's barley loaves, he fed thousands of people. "Jesus then took the loaves, gave thanks, and distributed to those ... as much as they wanted" (John 6:11).

Basil

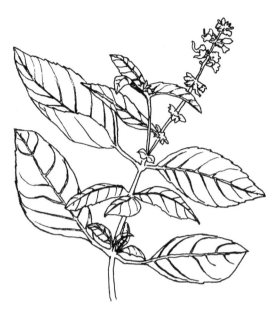

⊞ My all-time favorite because of its culinary and medicinal properties and aroma, of which I am particularly in favor. The Greeks seemed to feel the same way since the name is derived from their word for "king." Also known as St. Joseph's wort, referring to the kind Joseph of Arimethea, who buried Jesus' body in his own tomb. The plant has many varieties. A member of the mint family, but grown as an annual.

☼ Grows easily outside in the hot summer. In fact, with a little water it seems to flourish more in heat. I like to plant it among my tomato, pepper, and zucchini plants to help keep bugs away; and it reminds me that great Italian dishes will be coming. During the winter months, I grow it in the sunniest window in the house, along with other Italian favorites, oregano and parsley.

❦ Leaves and stems.

♡ Great for the digestive system. Stimulates the appetite and the bowels. Considered a worthy alternative to traditional headache medicines. Try a plate of pasta and pesto, instead of aspirin, next time you get a headache! I like to add freshly-cut herbs to my salad, as much as possible. Utilizing fresh herbs as an alternative to dressing enhances the flavor. Add cuttings of fresh herbs to white or red wine vinegar and allow them to flavor the vinegar. Olive oil, vinegar, and herbs are a great and healthy replacement for processed salad dressings.

♦♦♦ Utilize the essential oil for topical skin applications. Rub it on cuts, wounds, abrasions, insect bites and stings, and acne. It can be used as a rinse for oily hair.

🍽 Traditionally used for Italian and Mediterranean cooking—but don't limit it to that. I like to use basil in fresh salsas during the summer when tomatoes are in abundance or in place of lettuce on a sandwich or burger.

☞ Use the leaves, fresh or dried; but I like them better fresh.

📖 The children of God would use basil to strengthen them during times of fasting. Basil is also one of the bitter herbs used in the Passover meal.

❗ No cautionary concerns noted, although this is a strong herb.

Bay

(Bay Laurel, California Bay, Oregon Myrtle)

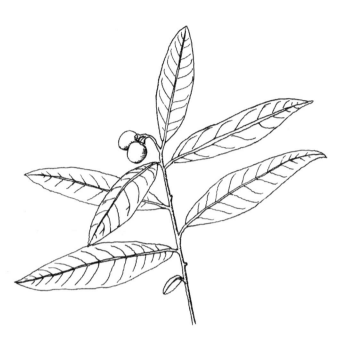

🏵 A beautiful and unique evergreen that can reach heights of 50 feet, producing white flowers that bloom in spring and develop into dark berries.

✿ Grows best in milder climates. I keep mine in a pot, sheltered during the winter months and it may grow slowly, 3 to 6 feet tall and is finicky. In its natural setting bay flourishes and spreads.

🌿 Leaves and the essential oils.

🝰 Said to have a calming and warming effect. Good for regulating digestion.

🛉🛉🛉 The essential oils are used in salves for treating rheumatism, bruises, and skin problems, and can be used to treat dandruff because of its astringent qualities.

🍽 Adds flavor to soup, stews, and pasta dishes, but before serving remove the leaves, which are not palatable, are hard to swallow, and don't digest.

📖 About the problem of evil, King David says, "I have seen a wicked and ruthless man flourishing like a green tree in its native soil, but he soon passed away and was no more" (Ps. 37:35-36).

In the land where I live, the bay tree flourishes and encroaches if not monitored, but it doesn't have a long life like a redwood or other trees. The reference David makes here is similar to the bay. He compares the evil person whose sinful lifestyle seems to go unpunished to the tree that grows and spreads so easily. It may seem as if the evil person's deeds go on unabated and without end; but soon he is gone like the morning mist. An evil life of 60 to 70 years doesn't compare with an eternity of judgment. Hitler did incredible damage and was as evil as could be, but his terrible reign only lasted a few years, and then he was gone, done in by his own hand. God will not let evil overrun his ultimate plan; and there will be no place for it in the blessed eternity awaiting us.

❗ Because it is an evergreen, bay has a caustic nature; so use moderately.

Bergamot

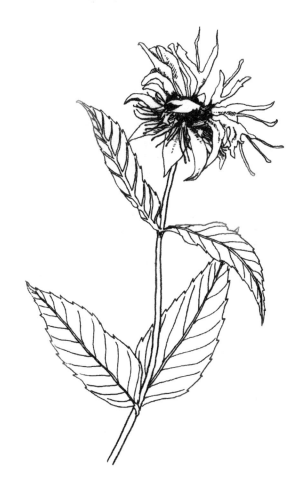

🏵 A hardy perennial found in many places of North America. A good garden plant, but does not tolerate real hot climates. Also known as monarda or horsemint, and as Oswego tea (because it is one of the substances used for tea during the colonial days of resistance to the tea tax). Its use remains popular today. Bergamot is sometimes confused with bee balm.

☼ This is a pretty garden plant that will attract butterflies and hummingbirds. These creatures love the flowers of white, pink, salmon and red hues. Bergamot grows similar to mint (although slower), so it can be invasive because of the spread of underground runners. Grows to heights of 2 to 3 feet. Highly aromatic.

�ு The leaves and the extracted oil.

📕 Like other mints, bergamot is a digestive aid that helps with heartburn, gas, and nausea. Bergamot may help with the symptoms of flu and chills. Native Americans in eastern areas were most familiar with this wonderful herb and used it for everything from headaches and backaches to a heart tonic.

👬 Old folklore suggests that, as a poultice, bergamot can be used to treat acne. Bergamot is great for aromatherapy. It is used in potpourri and dried bouquets. Or just enjoy it on a sunny day in the garden as the aroma rises around you.

🍵 A highly pleasant and fragrant flavor with a hint of mint. The leaves are used to flavor teas of all kinds, especially Earl Gray. Try a few new leaves mixed into a salad. Salad has never smelled so good.

☞ Use the leaves and flowers for teas and poultices. You can purchase oil of bergamot for a number of uses.

Berry
(Blackberry and Raspberry family)

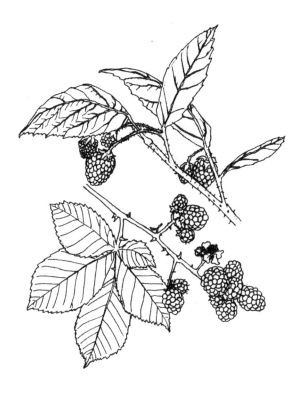

⊞ Thorny bushed plants produce an abundance of berries in the summer. They grow wild in abundance and are also grown and cultivated in the garden. I like to pick them wild in areas that haven't been sprayed heavily with pesticides and such. Long sleeves, long pants, and toed shoes make the picking safer.

✿ If you grow them on your property, just trying to keep up with them through pruning will be a challenge enough.

🌹 Leaves, stems, and berries.

🍵 High in fiber and vitamin C, these berries are naturally good for you picked fresh. But while you are at it, pick young tender leaves too, because they are great for herbal teas. Many manufacturers of herbal teas rely on berry leaves as a base for their teas. The leaves are beneficial for digestion and may help with diarrhea and nausea. It is said that red raspberry leaves help to tone uterine muscles before labor, help reduce labor pains, and help return the uterus to normalcy. Leaves are also said to increase milk production for lactating women.

👪 Berry juice can be used as a gargle for a sore mouth and throat, or for laryngitis. The leaves applied to the skin have an effect similar to aloe vera in soothing burns.

🍽 Many.

☞ Use the fruit, best fresh and in its most natural state. Use fresh leaves as a compress and dried leaves as a tea.

❗ For pregnant women: Use raspberry leaves only during the last two months of pregnancy, and only with your doctor's supervision.

24

Bilberry
(also Blueberry and Huckleberry)

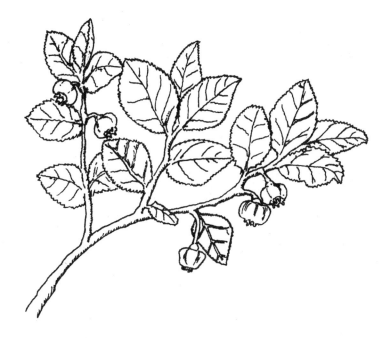

⚘ A deciduous shrub that prefers moist climates and non-alkaline soil. Plant does well in the same environment as rhododendrons and azaleas. There are many varieties of commercially-produced blueberries. Huckleberries are fun to pick in the wild. I have done so on the western slope of Mt. Adams in Washington. But be watchful! The bears like to pick and eat them, too.

✿ Prune the bushes to prevent overbearing; and to keep first-year plants from bearing, strip off flowers as they bloom.

🌿 Berries and leaves.

🗗 May improve night vision, eye strain and eye fatigue, stress, anxiety, vomiting, diarrhea, stomach cramps; and will help stabilize blood sugars, because it contains glucoquinine. The berries can cause diarrhea in some people and relieve it in others; so the benefits depend upon the individual's system. For inflammation in the mouth, gargling with the juice may help relieve symptoms. Leaf teas can be used for coughs and vomiting. Expect to see much more research done on these wonderful fruits in the years to come.

👫 Leaf tea can be used for skin disorders and for treating burns.

🍽 Great for jams, preserves, and jellies.

☞ Eat fresh; squeeze for juice; or boil 2 teaspoons dried leaves per cup of water.

❗ Excessive, continual use of the leaves may result in poisoning.

25

Blessed Thistle
(St. Benedict Thistle)

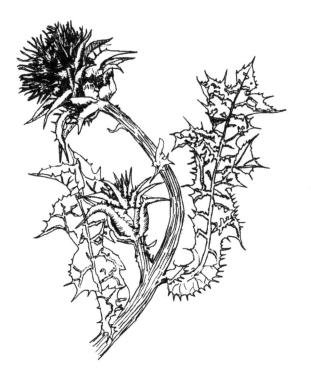

🏵 A member of the daisy family, this annual grows wild in some parts of North America. It has spiny leaves that sting, and it has a yellow flower that blooms throughout summer.

✿ No tips on growing; it's considered a weed.

🌿 The whole plant.

℧ Blessed thistle is used as an aid in improving digestion and relieving heartburn; regulate the menstrual cycle and help stimulate mother's milk production; plus strengthening the heart and liver. It's considered to have blood clotting properties. It's used to bring down high temperatures. Most interestingly, it's considered brain food that helps to stimulate the memory and combat depression.

☞ 1 teaspoon dried herb in ½ cup of water.

📖 The name is interesting enough in that the plant is named after St. Benedict, the founder of the order of the Benedictine monks. The herb's name is derived from the relationship between exorcism and this plant. Jesus, in Matthew 13:7, talks about the thorns and the thistles that overgrow the seeds a farmer plants. The purpose of the parable is to warn us that when we receive the Lord, we will want to keep out of our lives those things that will stunt or destroy our growth in him. Jesus was speaking to farmers who hated thorny weeds because they would be mixed with the harvest and they would injure their animals and themselves.

❗ No cautionary concerns noted. Just be careful of the stinging leaves.

Boneset

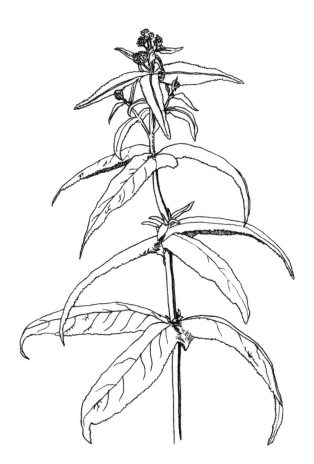

❁ Another North American perennial introduced to European immigrants by the Native Americans. If you are reading this during the cold and flu season, then this herb may be of some help. This plant is also known as "feverwort" among other names. The herb has a long hairy stem that can grow to 5 feet. Numerous small white flowers appear in the late summer and early fall. The name seems to come from the idea of breaking "bone fever" which was an influenza that had a hard effect upon early European Americans.

☼ This is a plant found in wetlands, so you need a moist area to grow it in. It can tolerate full sun but prefers some shade. The plant can be grown from seed or by dividing an existing plant.

🌿 The leaves, which have a bitter flavor, plus the flower.

🝢 Utilize boneset to relieve the stuffy-nose symptoms of colds and flu. You may find it effective for relieving coughs and respiratory congestion. True to one of its names, boneset may help reduce fever. You may also find that for constipation it can help and is said to have a calming effect upon the body.

☞ The leaves as a tea or in capsule form.

❗ Long-term use could result in toxicity.

Borage

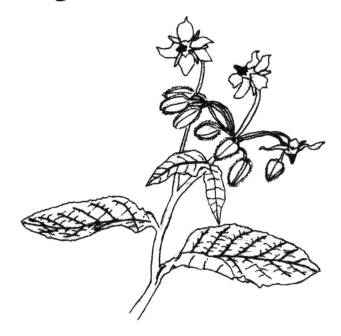

▦ An annual plant native to the Mediterranean that can grow to 2 feet tall. Borage has hairy leaves and stems and it bears purple, star-shaped flowers through the heat of summer.

☼ Treat as an annual that grows best after the last frost, but it will grow in any soil and likes the sun.

🌿 Leaves and flowers.

🗘 The herb's name suggests strengthening and the relieving of mild depression or the "blues." You can use it to boost your mood. People who have been ill for lengthy periods of time may find that borage works as a strengthening tonic. It also has a cooling and calming effect and may help break fevers.

It may have a healing effect upon people suffering from pleurisy. Borage contains gamma linoleic acid, which has been found to be helpful in treating PMS.

♦ The fresh herb has been used as an eyewash and for skin inflammations.

🍽 The flowers and the leaves can be used in iced teas and salads; you may notice a cucumber-like flavor.

☞ Use fresh; or dry the leaves and flowers.

❢ Extended use of borage is not recommended, and the leaves may cause dermatitis for people with very sensitive skin. And there is concern, because of alkaloids, that liver damage is possible if used in large amounts.

Burdock

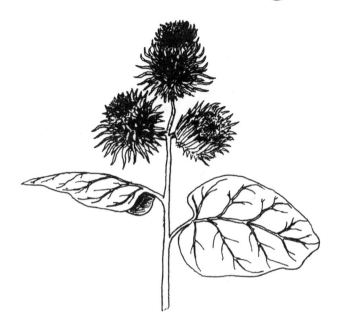

⊞ A biennial plant found in the northern parts of America. In its second year it may grow as tall as 3 feet, and you will note a reddish stem and woody branches. Purple flowers in clusters bloom July through September.

☼ Grows well in loose compost and soil.

�$ Root, seed, and leaves.

🗘 This herb is considered a blood purifier and a way to rid the body of harmful toxins. It has a diuretic action; so it will help to clean out the kidneys and urinary tract, and to lower blood pressure. Because of the diuretic properties, it may also help with arthritis, rheumatism, and even back pain caused from muscle strains.

🏘 Burdock can be used topically for eczema, psoriasis, acne, and canker sores. It may relieve the itch of poison oak and ivy. Using the leaves in an infusion also works as a skin tonic.

🍽 Some people like to use the root for soups, and for vegetable and meat dishes. The leaves and the stalks can be used in salads; or try using stalks, cooked, as you would asparagus.

☞ The root is the most-used part of the plant and, because of the above-mentioned concerns, is harvested in the second year in spring or fall. Use fresh leaves the first year. Grate the fresh root and add half the amount of water to ground root.

❣ Burdock can be constipating for some individuals.

Butcher's Broom

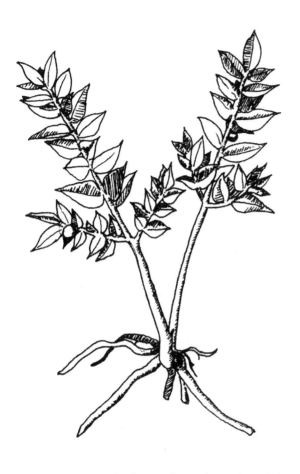

▣ An evergreen shrub, also known as "knee holly." Grows to 3 feet high and has greenish white flowers and red berries. In olden days, the fronds of butcher's broom were bound together and tied to a long stick to make a functional broom for sweeping out the butcher's shop; hence the name.

☼ Grows in most zones in the U.S.; likes more shade than sun. Spreads by underground stems and makes a unique ground cover plant.

❀ The whole herb.

℧ Best use is in the form of capsules or liquid from your local herb shop. If you are a person who has to be on your feet a lot, then this herb may make that task a little easier. This plant has some natural steroidal-type compounds. If you suffer from swelling of the legs and feet after a long day, or if you have restless leg syndrome, arthritis or rheumatism, then butcher's broom may be for you. You may also find that it helps relieve the symptoms of carpal tunnel syndrome, and improve circulation and vein structure in the hands and feet. This seems to be an herb with multiple uses, including helping to keep off excess body weight.

⚕ Salves and creams are made from this herb to help reduce the inflammation of hemorrhoids.

☞ Best uses are in capsule or oil form.

❗ If you have high blood pressure, then check with your doctor before taking butcher's broom.

Calendula

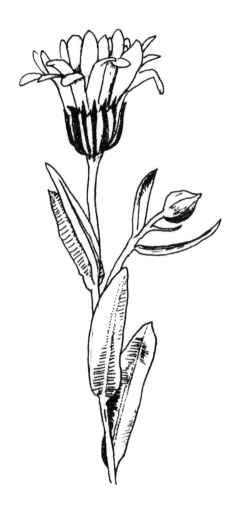

⚘ An annual plant that is very popular, grows 1 to 2 feet high, and blooms from spring to fall, depending upon the region in which you live. Produces lots of flowers in shades of yellow from apricot to cream. Also known as pot marigold. The name refers to a cooking pot, in that this is a culinary plant. But don't confuse it with traditional garden variety marigolds. Note the distinction, *Calendula officinalis*, before picking garden marigolds for herbal use.

☼ Sow in pots or directly in the ground after last frost. Likes lots of sun and doesn't need a lot of water. Pick off spent flowers to insure a steady bloom. If you live in a fairly mild climate without hard frosts, you may discover that you can grow this flower year round to give you beautiful orange and yellow blooms most of the year.

🌿 Leaves and flowers.

♍ Utilize the leaves, flowers, or derive the essential oil; taken orally it can help stem a fever, calm stomach cramps, ulcer, colitis, diarrhea, or help during a painful menstrual cycle.

⚕ The oil or a salve can help relieve the pain from burns, bruises, sprains, sore muscles, and even boils and shingles.

🍽 In the olden days, calendula was treated as a vegetable and used for cooking. If you want to try it, sprinkle some of the petals on a salad. You may note a bittersweet, salty flavor.

☞ Internally, use 1 teaspoon dried flowers per 1 cup water. Externally, use oil or use a commercially-made preparation.

❗ If you are pregnant, check with your doctor before using. This plant is not to be confused with the ever-popular African marigold, which is heavily sold in nurseries during the summer.

Carrot

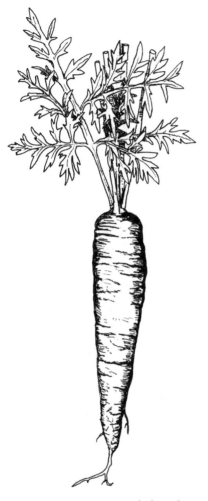

⊞ Bugs Bunny knows that the more of these vegetables, with great herbal qualities, he can get out of Elmer Fudd's garden, the better off he will be. This popular garden vegetable, which comes in many varieties, is very good for you.

✿ An easy plant to grow that does well in most climates, and, because it is an underground root, can often be grown year round in many climates. Sow seeds directly in well-cultivated soil with lots of room for root growth. I grow my carrots in large container boxes a foot deep. I scatter the seed and pull carrots for months, from little tender ones early in the season, to giant ones in the late fall. Even in the harsh climate where I live, carrots will often survive the winter.

⚘ Root and seed.

♉ Carrot is high in carotene, a natural form of vitamin A, which is a known cancer-fighter. Research has shown that consuming carrot and other vegetables high in carotene will help reduce your risk of getting certain types of cancer. Just one good-sized carrot per day will give you double the amount of recommended carotene. I was always told to eat carrots to prevent night blindness and to improve my eyesight; and there is proof that carrots help to increase the formation of visual purple.

Carrot consumption can help reduce coronary heart disease and lower blood cholesterol levels. Consumption can also help with heartburn, excess gas, and diarrhea. I like carrot juice, especially combined with other juices such as orange.

🍽 Many culinary uses. Good raw, cooked, or juiced.

☞ Eat and enjoy. What more can I say? But, the fresher, the better. And consume with the peel on. You can also make a tea of ground, wild carrot seed for digestive issues. The wild carrot root, however, is not very palatable. I have tried it. It's bitter. Wild carrot is also known as Queen Anne's lace because of its delicate white flower that blooms abundantly in some areas during summer. It is pretty to look at but the taste is just the opposite, not pretty, but bitter. If you are still interested in wild carrot, make sure that, when picking, and if you live in the midwest to the east, that you haven't picked poison hemlock, which looks similar.

Cascara Sagrada

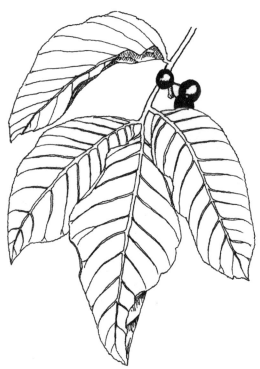

⌘ Also known as California buckthorn (*Rhamnus purshiana*), this is a deciduous evergreen tree that ranges in the mountainous areas of Northern California and also stretches east into Montana and north into Canada. Look for a tree growing up to 20-40 feet tall with reddish brown bark, dark green elliptical leaves, small greenish to white flowers, and a small black pea-sized fruit.

☼ A hardy tree that grows in most zones and is tolerant of deep shade to full sun if ample water is available. If you choose to grow one, you may enjoy its branching pattern and black berries.

🌹 The bark. (Also the berry can be consumed after being cooked and mashed.)

⛿ This is a purging herb considered a bitter herb in that its most common use is as a laxative. Native Americans have used this herb for centuries. It is believed that cascara sagrada bark is helpful with gallstones, liver concerns, and dyspepsia. This herb is widely distributed and is a good alternative to conventional laxatives which may be too strong on the body. This is a natural way to get normal bowel function, especially if you have been dealing with chronic constipation. Also, if you have a colon disorder or a parasitic infestation of the intestine or colon, cascara sagrada may be a great way to treat it with little or no harsh side effects. This seems to be God's version of "rotor rooter" for the bowels.

☞ The suggestion is to use aged bark, at least a year old. The dried bark is pulverized or ground into a powder. Mix one teaspoon of powder with 1½ cups of very hot water. After the liquid cools, then drink it. This can be made into a tea or a tincture, however it has a very bitter taste, so you may choose to opt for capsules that can be purchased at your local health food store.

❗ Overuse could cause cramps and diarrhea because of the bitter nature of the leaves. This herb acts as a stimulant on the bowels, so too much could cause overstimulation. However, that is the case with most laxatives, and cascara sagrada is one of the safest and most natural laxatives you can use.

Castor Bean

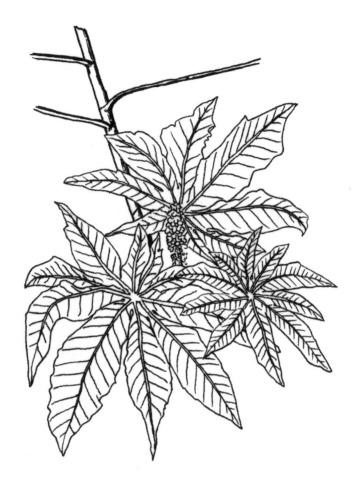

🏵 A huge leafy plant that can grow in excess of 10 feet. Large, but poisonous seeds, large lobed leaves that can reach a size of 2½ feet with small white flowers. Grown as an annual but in milder climates it can winter over and continue on for many years. My generation, the baby boomers, and certainly my parent's depression-era generation are all too familiar with the bitter taste of castor oil. Fortunately there are now better options. I include this herb only because of its familiarity and its biblical links. And it may be the poisonous gourd mentioned in 2 Kings 4:38-40 which hears men crying out, "O man of God, there is death in the pot!" Elisha the prophet made the stew safe for the men to eat. Let that be a warning of the danger of this plant.

☼ Makes an interesting ornamental, so don't be surprised to see your neighbor growing one. Needs lots of space, sun and water. Because of the plant's toxicity I don't recommend that you grow it where small children could possibility ingest it.

🌹 The oil pressed and carefully processed from the seeds.

🗁 A strong purgative for acute constipation that has lost favor in recent years because of its harshness.

🍽 None. This is a toxic plant that is to be handled carefully.

☞ I would only use castor oil under a doctor's care and strictly as prescribed. Castor oil is not readily available as it was a generation or two ago because there are other options and alternatives. See cascara sagrada for a safer alternative.

📖 It is believed by Bible scholars that this is the plant under which the petulant Jonah sat and received comforting shade. "Then the Lord God provided a vine and made it grow up over Jonah to give shade for his head to ease his discomfort and Jonah was very happy about the vine" (Jonah 4:6). The prophet Jonah had already spent 3 days in the belly of a large fish for not doing what God wanted him to do, then he had carried out the mission but remained unhappy. He went to evil Ninevah and prophesied that if the people didn't turn away from their wicked ways Jehovah would destroy them. Then he was mad because they *did* turn their hearts to God. Seems selfish? But aren't we all that way now and then? We have our expectations about how God should act and then when he doesn't do as we think he should we become perplexed, disappointed, and irritated. But that is exactly the problem. Jonah had reason to not want to see Ninevah saved; they had persecuted his people for ages. He thought, why should mercy be extended to them? But the reality is: how much have we tortured God by *our* ways? And yet *we* expect mercy.

How do we deal with such disappointing and perplexing situations? We need to realize that through human eyes we see through "a glass darkly," and "God's ways are higher than ours." Resorting to our value system we shortchange God who knows infinitely more about the situation. Compared to God, we only truly have an iota's worth of wisdom and knowledge about things. We can participate in God's great plan or we can pout in our own futility. But then think about that, see the glass half full and take some comfort there. I don't have to know everything, I just need to live in the mustard seed of faith that he has given me and seek to carry out what he desires in the knowledge that perfect God knows perfectly best. Let him worry about the big stuff. I just need to concern myself with those for whom I take responsibility: family, others in need, and myself. Jonah found momentary comfort from the heat of the day in the giant leaves of the castor bean plant, but we can do better and enjoy the shade and protection of God's hand as we hide there. "He hideth my soul in the depths of his love and covers me there with his hand."

❗ Many cautionary concerns. This is a strong purgative that is not only harsh on the bowel system but can have an adverse effect upon the heart and kidneys. The deadly poison, ricin is made from a derivative of castor bean. This is another good reminder to us of the curse under which we live. Here is a plant that has good properties, that provided cooling shade for Jonah, but that also has within its properties a substance that will kill you.

Catnip
(Catmint)

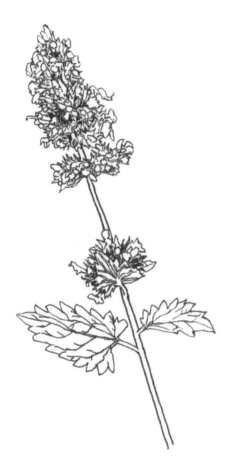

⊞ A member of the mint family grown as a perennial. Unlike most mints, catnip grows to heights of 5 feet. A gray-green color with fine downy hairs on its stalks, catnip has an abundance of white and purple flowers; doesn't have the pleasant aroma of most mints and is not a particularly attractive plant; imported from Europe; grows wild. Catnip's scientific name is *Nepeta Cateria* and catmint's scientific name is *Nepeta Faassenii.*

☼ Seeds are readily available but you may be able to divide roots of an existing plant. I suggest you keep it in a container or plant it in the ground in the container with the bottom removed. That will help prevent spreading and encroaching. Don't be surprised if the neighborhood cats take a greater interest in your garden. Grow a small amount, see what you think. One fellow indicated the plant smelled like dirty socks, so you may want to find a far corner of your garden. In Europe the plant was grown to keep rats and mice out of the garden.

🌷 The flowering tops and leaves as a tea.

🗘 It may drive your cat crazy. But if you use it, it will probably have just the opposite effect on you. Catnip is a calming, safe, and mild sedative. It seems to help the digestive system with gas, indigestion, stomach discomfort, and diarrhea. You may find it helps in relieving symptoms of bronchitis. This plant is called field balm because of its warming and comforting effect upon mind and body. And it may help with headaches, fevers and chills, and the achy conditions that go with them. Catnip tea or capsules from your health food store could be part of your arsenal during cold and flu season.

👬 Try fresh leaves in a bath.

🍽 In France the plant is utilized as a seasoning.

☞ The leaves made into a tea, 1 teaspoon with 1 cup hot, not boiling, water.

❗ This is a very safe herb that you could even give to a colicky child.

Cayenne
(Capsicum)

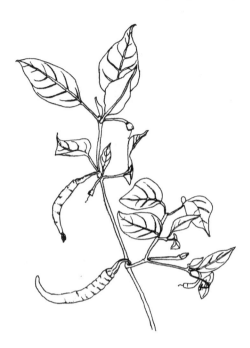

The chili pepper is the most commonly used source of cayenne, but there are many varieties of hot peppers. and there are many benefits other than just the fun of eating something so spicy.

☼ Other than in southwest desert areas, it does best in the hottest part of summer and is grown as an annual. May grow to 6 feet tall. White blossoms mature into red and yellow fruit. Very susceptible to frost, so plant outside only after there is no possibility of frost. Where I live, late frost is a danger. I start the plants in pots, then transplant later. Grow in the sunniest part of the garden and water conservatively.

The fruit.

Surprisingly, this herb that burns your mouth is a tonic for the stomach and bowels. A general digestive aid that increases gastric juices and boosts metabolism. Full of vitamin B complex, vitamin C, iron, and calcium, it's said to ward off colds. So stoke up on peppers as cold and flu season nears. Cayenne stimulates the brain by kicking endorphins into high gear. Consumption of the pepper may increase feelings of ease, as well as lower cholesterol and reduce headaches. Makes you want some hot, spicy salsa, doesn't it? Well, eat and enjoy your way to better health.

A liniment of cayenne may help relieve arthritis and rheumatism pain.

Many and varied culinary uses. Have at it. Try it in a variety of foods. Dice and add to scrambled eggs, tuna sandwiches, or baked potatoes.

Other than general consumption, or if your mouth is too sensitive, capsules are available at most health food stores. Make a tea using ½ to 1 teaspoon ground cayenne to 1 cup boiling water.

None noted, but I couldn't help but think of this. James Chapter 3 warns us to tame the tongue. Our words issued off our tongue can be biting and hot as the pepper or as soothing as a cup of chamomile tea. James says the tongue can be like a fire, setting the course of a life on its way to hell. Is our talk peppered with vulgarity, rumor, dissension? Or do our words offer strength and light to those who struggle in darkness and despair? We have the choice.

Cayenne can agitate sensitive skin and body areas. I once got a little in my eye and it bothered me for hours. Prolonged use on the skin can raise blisters. Cayenne can aggravate hemorrhoids. Excessive use can cause kidney damage.

Celery

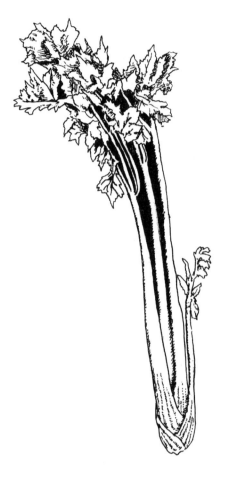

▦ A common garden vegetable. A biennial that may survive winters in some zones. Grows wild in some parts of North America, in more alkaline soils.

☼ Prefers damp and rich soil. Fertilize every 2 to 3 weeks. In milder climates, try starting the plant in summer to grow as a winter crop. Watch for snails and slugs, because they will enjoy the plant before you get to.

❧ Roots, leaves, juice, and seeds.

♄ Right after you enjoy a hot pepper, crunch on a celery stalk to help chase the sting away. Herbalist John Lust believes that the expressed juice is the most effective part of the plant. It can be used for dropsy, rheumatism, and gout; to maintain or lose weight; to treat gas and pulmonary problems. Celery is a diuretic; it may help keep kidneys in tone and lower high blood pressure. It is said to help regulate the menstrual process and improve skin. The seeds are said to be good for bronchitis. They also have a calming effect on nerves and stress.

🍽 Certainly the obvious ones. Because celery has sodium in it, try sprinkling ground or whole celery seed instead of salt. You will get the benefits of salt as well as the additional benefits of celery.

☞ As a decoction or tea, use ½ teaspoon seeds to ½ cup water, boil briefly and then strain. As an essential oil, use a few drops twice a day. As a juice, mix 1 or 2 tablespoons with carrot or apple juice.

📖 None noted, but it is often used as one of the bitter herbs in Passover feasts as a reminder of the bitterness of bondage. Here is a thought: What holds you in bondage? If you are considering changing your diet for the better, then perhaps you are considering coming out of a bondage of misuse to your body. Because you are probably familiar with celery, its consumption is an easy way to begin that process.

❗ Some sources suggest that because of the high salt content, you should be careful if you already have high blood pressure. If you are pregnant, avoid the juice or oil.

Chamomile

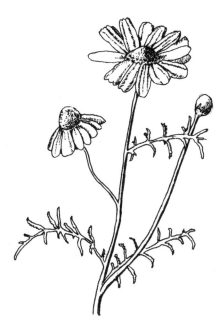

✖ A member of the daisy family with small white and yellow flowers. Feathery, delicate leaves. This pretty plant looks good in garden or flower pot. Outside, the plant dies each year, but re-seeds and spreads. Easy to control, though, and has a wonderful aroma—sweet, but not as strong as many herbs. An all-time favorite I use nearly every day.

✿ Easy to grow, but has very small seeds. Place shallow in well-cultivated, rich soil in spring. Likes sun. Numerous varieties. Europeans use short-growing varieties as an alternative to traditional grass lawn.

🌹 The flowers.

🍵 As one who has sleep struggles, I like a commercially-produced herbal tea called "Sleepy Time" that contains chamomile. After a hectic day, this soothing and fragrant tea relaxes me and helps me nod off to sleep. Recommended for stress and anxiety relief. Chamomile is thought to stimulate serotonin in the brain, beneficial for a sense of well-being, and may help in the reduction of pain and depression. Has been proven to aid in the healing of the stomach wall and intestines if they become ulcerated. Once I was attacked by a bacteria that kept me ill for months. I believe the regular use of chamomile put me on the road to recovery by helping to heal my tortured digestive system. Having a warm cup of chamomile tea is like drinking a fragrant flower garden. One of the best all-purpose and safe herbs.

👥 Good for skin disorders, sore joints, swellings, even hemorrhoids. Can be used as a mouth wash and to help relieve a toothache. Blond persons may discover the oil of essence will enhance their golden appearance.

🍽 Sprinkle flower petals on salads.

☞ Harvest flowers at their peak. Tie into bundles and hang in a warm, dry area. The wonderful fragrance will fill the room. Use dried flowers liberally in teas. Also tuck some into a pillow or in a clothes drawer.

📖 None found. But the gentle plant reminds me of the grace Jesus Christ offers. He said, "Peace I leave with you; my peace I give you" (Jn. 14:27). This peace surpasses understanding and gives assurance that, while the world wages war and discontent, all is well between God and me because of Christ's sacrifice. He has overcome the world for me. Tonight, enjoy a cup of chamomile tea while reading a Psalm.

❗ Very safe herb. Only a concern if you are allergic to flowers of the daisy family.

Chicory

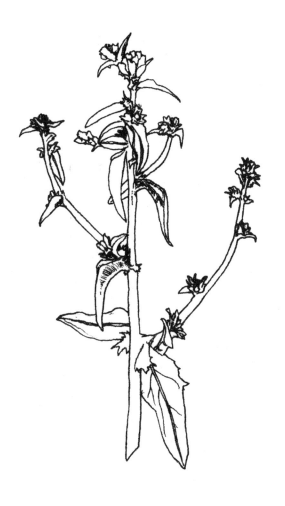

▣ A perennial plant that grows wild in America. If you found it growing in your yard, you would consider it a weed. The plant looks similar to the wildflower "bachelor button." The plant grows 2 to 3 feet tall, and it has light blue to violet-blue flowers that bloom summer to fall.

☼ To grow chicory in your garden, you will want to place the plant where it can develop the deep root system it needs. It is the root you will harvest for many uses. Confine the plant to one contained area, because it will spread. I have grown it in deep pots.

🌾 Rootstock and flowers.

☕ If your stomach can't handle coffee anymore, then chicory may be for you. Many coffee substitutes have chicory as a main ingredient.

Chicory is also said to be helpful for liver and spleen problems and in treating jaundice. It may be helpful for gastritis and digestive problems. The benefits of this plant are similar to those of dandelion.

👫 Native Americans also have used it as a topical compress for swellings and inflammations.

🍽 You will find chicory in many herbal tea blends available at stores, so if you are an herbal tea lover, then you are probably already consuming chicory. You can also add the young leaves or flowers to a salad.

☞ The rootstock is gathered in the spring and dried and can be ground. Leaves and flowers can be used as a poultice for external uses such as inflammations.

Chive

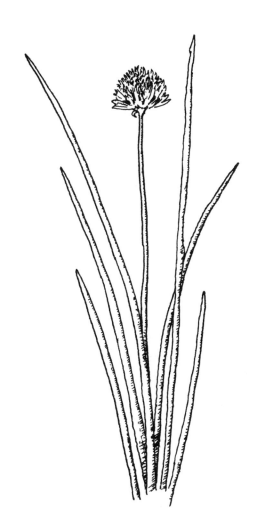

⊞ A perennial related to the onion, the chive plant grows to a height of at least 12 inches with small onion-like stems and onion smell. The plant blooms a large blue or purple flower on a tall stem that lasts for a long time. Then once the bloom is gone, you have many seeds for planting.

✿ Chives make a great addition to the flower garden because of the pretty and unique flowers. The plant acts as an insect repellent so it will help keep the bugs away. I grow chives in pots year round, and in a sunny location in the house during the winter months. You can find garlic chive seeds available and this is a great addition to your herb garden. In fact, I prefer these to any other because of their great taste, texture, and aroma.

🌱 The onion-like stems and the flowers.

☡ Chive, like onion, promotes good digestion and regularity. It contains iron, so it is good for anemia. It is also high in vitamin C, so it is a unique way to get that needed vitamin, if you don't want citrus.

🍽 Chop fresh and sprinkle on salads, soups, and baked potatoes. I like to put chives in fresh salsa and in scrambled eggs or omelets.

☞ Fresh is best. While dried chive is available in the spice section of grocery stores, much of the value has been lost in the drying process.

❗ Use caution if you are iron-sensitive.

Cinnamon
(Cassia)

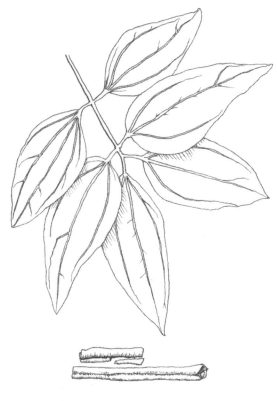

🏵 Two types are most familiar: *Cinnamomum Verum*, or true cinnamon and *Cassia*, or Chinese cinnamon. For table use, we are more familiar with Chinese cinnamon. Both herbs come from the bark of the cinnamon trees. Chinese cinnamon is much more pungent and bitter. Both trees are evergreen and related to laurel.

✿ Many varieties of *Cassia*, used as ornamentals, are related to cinnamon and are available at nurseries.

🌿 The inner bark and the extracted oil.

♉ Aids digestion, helps relieve diarrhea and nausea; counteracts congestion and eases symptoms of common cold. Cinnamon assists in improving circulation. It's a warming herb that could also help with the metabolism of fats. It's an effective agent in the fight against fungus. Cinnamon is helpful for treating the symptoms of diabetes, yeast infections, and uterine hemorrhaging.

💮 The smell of cinnamon is a soothing aromatherapy in perfumes and incense. Cinnamon is added to ingredients for shampoo. The Song of Solomon speaks of the lover's garden (a double entendré) being filled with such fragrances as cinnamon.

🍽 This is such a commonly used herb/spice that you can doubtless tell *me* all the things it could be used for. But it's nice to know something as simple as cinnamon toast may help digestive problems and offer some relief for colds.

☞ Try cinnamon bark, and grind it yourself for a more fresh taste.

📖 Cinnamon and *Cassia* have numerous mentions in the Bible. This wonderful herb or spice was highly favored. King Solomon may have cultivated the trees. Exodus 30:22 describes it as one of the ingredients for the anointing oil used in the temple. Oil symbolizes the Holy Spirit. The next time you get a pleasant whiff of cinnamon, let it remind you of the wonderful work the Holy Spirit does in you to make you a fragrant offering in your service and worship to the Lord.

❗ Seems to be a very safe herb. But cinnamon in tea gives people like me heartburn.

Clover

(Red) Wild Clover

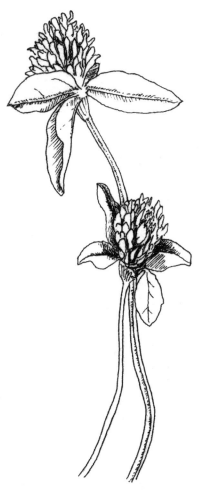

▣ You have probably seen this lawn-like perennial in many places in North America. Red clover is unique because of its reddish stems.

☼ Grows abundantly in the wild and probably has encroached into your yard. Makes an effective ground cover that will help hold inclines and banks.

❧ The whole plant, but especially the flowering tops.

♈ This herb acts as a muscle relaxer. It is also used as an expectorant. Helps treat skin problems and inflammations, from eczema to athlete's foot. Red clover combined with other herbs may actually help to shrink cancerous tumors. Red clover is an overall body tonic that aids in digestion disorders from top to bottom. It has been recently used in treating HIV and AIDS because it is believed to help boost a weakened immune system.

ﬔ As a poultice or oil, for rheumatism and gout.

🍽 Use fresh in salads.

☞ As a kid I would pick it and eat the flowers and leaves on the spot, though I didn't realize it was good for me. The leaves and flowers can also be used as a tea or a poultice.

📖 The three-leaf clover was significant to early Christians who saw the triune God, or the Trinity in its shape. But if they were "lucky" enough to find a four-leaf clover, then those early Christians thought not about luck, but the cross. The four leaves were a reminder to them of the cross and the cost God paid for them. Think about it the next time you look at one of the clovers; is this not a great living parable? For some, the concept of the triune nature of God is hard to understand. Represented in the clover is a picture of this triple aspect of this God Who is One. Here is one leaf with three separate parts, yet all joined together. Then consider the rare "four leaved" clover—this God loved us so much that he would die for us so he could be joined with us. What god would die for his beloved except the One True God who would not live without us?

Clove Tree

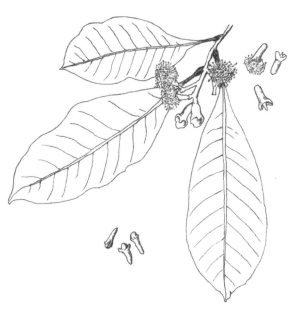

✤ A deciduous ever-green tree native to Indonesia and such places as the Philippines, Sumatra, West Indies and some countries of South America. Grows to heights of 30 feet with long leaves of up to 5 inches and red and white bell-shaped flowers.

☼ This is a tropical plant; so if you were to grow one you would have to have that type of climate or grow it indoors much of the year, provide high humidity, and have temperatures that never drop below 60 degrees.

▽ The most common use is the oil of clove for immediate relief of a toothache. A generation ago, no household would be without cloves. I can remember feeling instant relief from a toothache on a weekend when I couldn't get to a dentist. Clove-flavored chewing gum gives spicy fresh breath. A few drops of oil of clove in water is said to help a queasy, nauseated digestive system.

♈ As an antiseptic clove is used as one ingredient in natural soaps and shampoos. As aromatherapy it's used in incense and scented candles.

🍽 Spice up desserts, hams, pickles, soups, etc. Remember, a little goes a long way.

☞ By crushing the dry flower buds or the extracted oil.

📖 No biblical reference noted, but certainly it was one of the many spices traded and used in perfumes, etc. This highly aromatic spice could have been one of the substances utilized in the anointing of the Lord and then also in the embalming of his body. In the anointing the pleasing aroma announced and signified the pleasing nature of God to give us his Son. In death, it masked the stench.

As Christians we too are to be a pleasing aroma. "But thanks be to God, who always leads us in triumphal procession in Christ and through us spreads everywhere the fragrance of the knowledge of him. For we are to God the aroma of Christ among those who are perishing. To one we are the smell of death; to the other, the fragrance of life" (2 Cor. 2:14-15). Some will reject the message and die in their sins and some will receive the message and live. Either way, as in the anointing or in the burial of Christ, the aroma remains pleasant.

❗ Be aware that pure clove oil is very strong and can cause irritation, so cut it with olive oil or water before use.

Cocoa
(Cacao or Chocolate)

This and the following two "herbs" I include in this new edition because numerous people ask me, almost with a pleading tone, "Can't chocolate, or cola or coffee be considered herbs?!" Well, here is the lowdown on these desirable but questionable herbal uses. With this information, I'll leave you to judge for yourself.

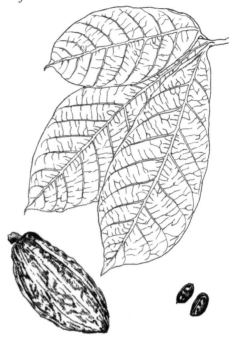

⊞ The term *Theobroma cacao*—chocolate fiends will be happy to hear—means "Food of the gods." The Mexican culture has given us the name 'chocolate.' The cacao tree grows to 16 feet with bright green leaves, small reddish colored flowers, and a yellowish- to red-colored fruit in which we get the seeds that are ground to make cocoa and chocolate. The tree is ever-bearing in leaves and bears fruit year round.

☼ This tropical plant needs a tropical climate plus some shade. In the wild and in orchards, cacao is usually an under-story tree with larger trees growing around it to provide shade.

⚘ The roasted seeds.

⛉ Cocoa in its raw form works as a diuretic and will help lower blood pressure, and because of this some tout chocolate as a heart tonic.

� Cocoa is a great emollient for skin and is helpful in reducing the noticeable presence of wrinkles.

🍽 Many—and how about s'mores!

☞ To use medicinally, you will need to find a source that provides the powder.

📖 None noted. However, when I discovered that the cacao tree grows fruit continuously, I couldn't help but think of the Tree of Life that will grow along the banks of the River of Life in Heaven, producing fruit continuously, a fruit that will be "for the healing of the nations." (See Ez. 47:12 and Rev. 22:2.)

❗ I must admit that I can do without the caffeine of colas and coffees, but chocolate is another story. Hey, we each have a weakness; chocolate is mine. However, the fact that I like it doesn't answer the question, Is chocolate good for you? It's unlikely, considering the way it is processed, and with all the sugar added. There certainly seems to be some benefit to the cacao seed, specifically for the skin, but by the time it's processed into cocoa and chocolate the minimal health benefits are often overshadowed by the additives. So, does that mean I am not going to enjoy chocolate any more? No!

Coffee

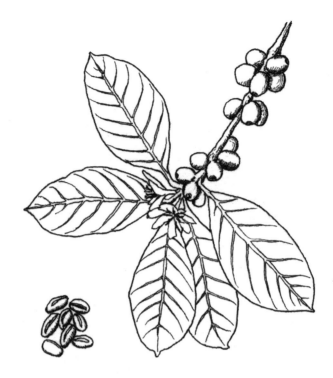

⊞ *Coffea Arabica*, native to East Africa, grows to heights of 15 feet. The name coffee seems to come from the word 'caffa' which was a province of Abyssinia. This is an attractive plant with 6-inch long leaves and small fragrant white flowers. The flowers are followed by ½ inch fruit that start green and gradually turn purple or red. Inside the fruit are two seeds, the coffee beans.

☼ This is a tropical plant that is very sensitive to cool temperatures and the lack of a high humidity. It can be grown as an ornamental house plant. I grew one once. The tree needs shade. Use mixes and fertilizers formulated for camellias.

🌺 The roasted seeds.

♉ If there is a medical use, then maybe as a diuretic. But there doesn't seem to be much benefit to the caffeine.

🍽 Many, but none noted in my herbal research.

☞ The grinding of the bean or seed.

❗ There are plenty of cautionary concerns, not that it matters to coffee drinkers. Caffeine is not good for you, and because the beverage acts as a diuretic, the more coffee you drink, the more dehydrated you will become. It also is said that it weakens the urinary tract and the bowels. Certainly God gave us the coffee bean; maybe we just haven't found the best use for it yet?

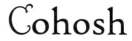

Cohosh

Blue & Black

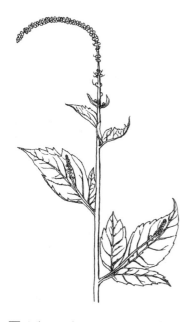

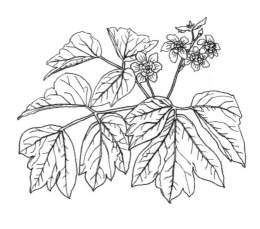

⊞ These plants are native from midwestern to eastern North America. Black cohosh is a large plant that can produce a stem reaching to heights of 7 to 9 feet. Leaves are oblong and the small white flowers grow in long bunches. It's also known as "black snakeroot" because it was used to treat snake bite. While black cohosh lives in ravines and mountain sides, though, blue cohosh prefers wetlands and riparian habitats. Look for six-pointed yellowish-green flowers with a pea-sized fruit.

✿ Seeds are available, and the plants can be propagated by splitting the roots or rhizomes. Cohosh prefers partial shade and rich, well-drained soil. The dried seed clusters are attractive for dried flower arrangements. You may not enjoy the aroma or odor of the black cohosh, however.

❦ The rootstalk of both plants.

✇ This plant has recently been "discovered" for its women's-health possibilities. The herb is said to help induce menstruation and relieve menstrual cramps. It is said to help women in labor and delivery. But this plant isn't just for women. It is helpful with respiratory conditions—everything from coughs to asthma and bronchitis. The plant is said to help with muscle spasm and symptoms of rheumatism, and to be an over-all tonic for jittery nerves because of its tranquilizing properties.

✦ None noted. Blue cohosh can irritate the skin.

☞ The rootstock, which is to be gathered in the fall after the leaves have died. However, safest use may be to purchase processed herb from your health store.

❗ Black cohosh is very strong and overuse could be poisonous. The berries in blue cohosh can be poisonous. The plant can irritate your skin upon contact. These are herbs that should be used only after consulting a medical authority and may be best in processed form, such as capsules or powder, bought at a health store.

Cola

(Kola Tree)

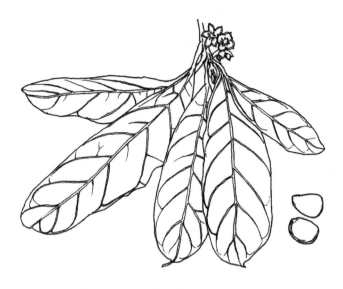

⊕ *Cola acuminata* is originally from West Africa but is now grown as a crop in South America and the West Indies. The kola nut is grown and harvested for the bitter, yellow-to-brown pods that carry the white or red nuts.

☼ This is a tropical plant needing tropical conditions to be grown in the states.

🌿 The roasted seeds.

♉ As a stimulant, because of the caffeine it contains. Cola seeds actually have more caffeine in them than coffee beans have. But my wife will tell you nothing gets rid of a headache quicker. She also might tell you, at three in the morning, "I can't sleep!"

👪 None noted.

🍽 The seeds are used as a seasoning in Western and Central tropical Africa. That tradition was picked up by the peoples of the West Indies and Brazil.

☞ Powder from the kola nut.

❗ Like coffee, it is the caffeine that is the problem, and so it will cause similar problems. And because we add sweeteners to this bitter herb, plus lots of other additives, then this stuff becomes a health risk. Some professionals are concerned that obesity and the rise in adult diabetes may be partially blamed on the increased consumption of soft drinks.

As requested, I have included these last three herbs. But as you may easily discern, there seems to be little benefit, at least in the way they are currently being consumed. That doesn't mean there won't be new discoveries of better uses for them. And it probably doesn't mean that in minimal moderation you can't enjoy these herbs in the products in which they are utilized, every once in a while. But maybe we should consider this, and make it a matter of prayer: "Lord, does my use of these products affect my need to be in your perfect will?"

Columbine

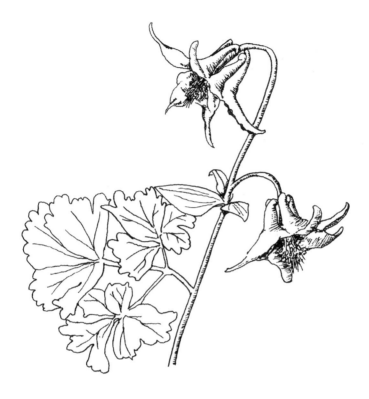

⊞ Here is one of my favorites in the garden because of its unique, wildflower look. A perennial that will come back in spring in most zones of the U.S., the plant can grow to 2½ feet high, depending upon the variety you grow. Columbine will blossom unique flowers of lavender and white during spring and early summer. Numerous varieties are being developed from this European transplant. Columbine is the state flower of Colorado.

✿ Grows easily enough in many climates. Place it in a pot or in a permanent place outdoors; water and fertilize normally; and the plant should do well.

🌿 Flowers, stems, and root.

🗗 Tea from the root is said to help with symptoms of diarrhea.

👪 As a topical astringent in a salve for rheumatism.

🍽 The flowers can be used to decorate a salad.

☞ As a tea, 1 teaspoon of plant parts in 1 cup water.

❗ No cautionary concerns noted. Uses for columbine are limited, but it is such a pretty and unique flower, I wanted to mention it here. Also, you may find that the hummingbirds will enjoy columbine's internal benefits more than you will.

Comfry

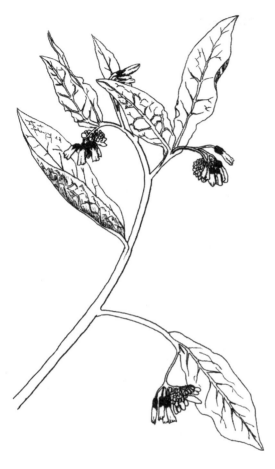

⊞ A perennial meadow plant growing 2-4 feet tall. Plant has black roots, tongue-shaped leaves with white to lavender tube-shaped flowers that bloom from early summer to early fall.

✿ Grow carefully, as this plant can overrun a garden. If you grow one for the rootstock or just to say you have one as part of your herb collection, then contain it in a large pot.

🕸 The sap from the root stock is the medicinal part.

✆ At one time comfry was used to treat stomach and bowel problems but there has been some concern and study done regarding the possibility of developing liver cancer because of comfry use. Comfry is banned in some countries.

ᵐ Treats skin irritations, insect bites and wounds and because of the presence of allantoin, comfry may even stimulate new cell growth. Comfry is added to commercially-prepared skin care products. Poultices and such may even help with soothing and repairing damaged tendons and ligaments.

🍽 None noted. Not recommended.

☞ Use as prepared powders, poultices, ointments and salves; or use the rootstock in baths.

❗ At this point, by the experts, not considered safe for internal or external use by pregnant or nursing mothers.

50

Coriander

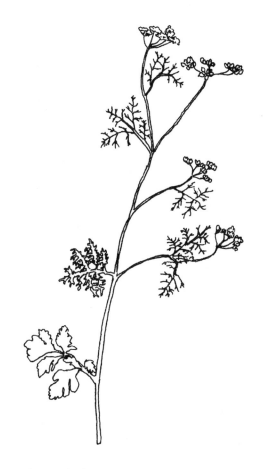

🏵 A small, annual plant with thin stems that grows 1 to 2 feet tall. During the heat of the summer months, white to reddish flowers appear in compound umbels. Coriander seeds have an unpleasant smell until they ripen.

☼ See tips on anise.

🌾 The seed. After it has ripened, it is picked and then dried.

☞ Considered a stomach aid. Coriander is said to be good for rheumatism and arthritis. It has been considered, by some, an aphrodisiac.

👫 Ground seed, mixed into a paste, can be applied to areas where rheumatism has set in, or on painful joints.

🍽 Highly-favored as a flavoring for many foods.

☞ Coriander seed is dried after it has ripened and been picked.

📖 When the nation of Israel was in route from Egypt to the Promised Land, God blessed them with a food source called "manna." Delivered miraculously each morning, this heavenly substance sustained the Hebrews. Exodus Chapter 16 tells us that manna compared in taste to coriander and the sweetness of wafers made with honey. Therefore, coriander is a good reminder to us that God supplies our needs daily. The Hebrew women would grind the manna into a flour and bake bread with it. What did Jesus tell us to pray for as part of the Lord's prayer? "Give us this day our daily bread." But Jesus also said that, "Man does not live on bread alone, but on every word that comes from the mouth of God" (Lk. 4:4).

Cranberry

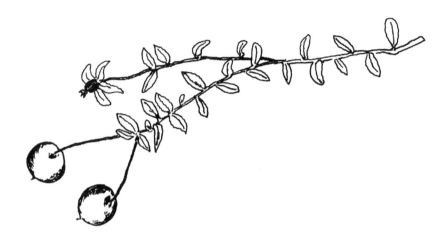

⊞ The plant that produces the dark red berries popular at Thanksgiving and Christmas time.

☼ Normally grown commercially in bogs and usually in coastal conditions. Both the northeast and the northwest coasts grow tons of cranberries for commercial use. There are varieties that grow well in other climates. I grow an American cranberry variety successfully in the high desert land of Oregon, where I live.

❀ The berry.

⚘ At one time, most of us only ate cranberries in highly-processed forms. Now, many of us drink the juice on a more regular basis. Research has shown that cranberry is very beneficial for kidney and urinary function, and in helping to prevent cystitis. It is possible the juice and oils keep bacteria from collecting in the bladder.

🍽 As a relish and as a juice. But seek ways to prepare cranberries without all the sugar, such as combining with pure apple juice. Or cook with honey for sauce.

☞ Cranberry in capsule form is available at most health food stores and pharmacies that carry herbal supplements.

❗ For people unaccustomed to eating healthily and utilizing herbs, cranberry can cause heartburn.

Cucumber

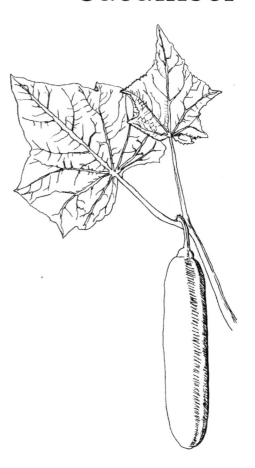

⬛ The common fruit of the cucumber plant. There are many varieties of plants to choose from. You may just think of this as a garden vegetable used in salads and made into pickles. But many vegetables and fruits have herblike healing qualities, and so qualify as herbs. Plus, there is a spiritual reference here. So have a pickle while you read this section, and enjoy!

🌹 The fruit.

👌 Cucumber works as a mild diuretic, helping to cleanse the body and eliminate excess water and other harmful accumulations like uric acid, kidney and bladder stones. Cucumber is beneficial for the kidneys and the heart and could have a positive effect upon blood pressure. Cucumber juice benefits the intestines, lungs, and skin. Research suggests that a property in cucumber may help keep cholesterol in check.

🏥 Many dermatologists and cosmetologists utilize cucumber for soothing and rejuvenating the skin. Evidently, Cleopatra used it on her skin, and we all know the effect she had on men.

🍽 A salad of cucumbers, plus tomatoes, onions, and herbs such as basil, mixed with olive oil and vinegar will help in a very delicious way to keep your bowels regular.

☞ For external purposes, extract the juice and use it fresh.

📖 The nation of Israel complained to Moses about not having cucumbers as they traveled to the Promised Land. God, in turn, mourned about his people in Isaiah 1:8. Their disobedience and rebelliousness weighed heavily on him and he compares them to the evil ones that lived in Sodom and Gomorrah. In our life with God, he asks us not to look back with longing at the things we used to have, because the old ways and the new way do not blend. God wants us to rely upon him wholly and to, in faith, be willing to step out for a new journey and a better place. He promises us that he will give us a life that is abundant. The things of the old life will pale in comparison to what he will provide for us.

❗ No cautionary concerns noted, but some people do get heartburn from eating this vegetable.

Dandelion

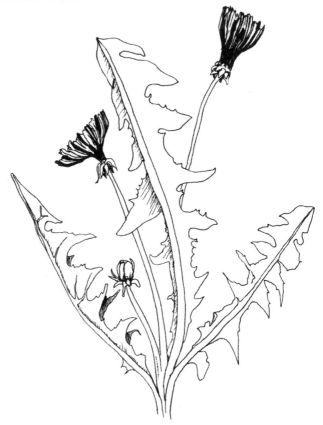

🏵 Yep, that weed! The one you do all you can to irradicate from your lawn each spring. The one with the bright yellow flower that reminds you of a lion's mane. And this is the one the kids like to pick in little bouquets for mom.

☼ "You're kidding, right?" I can hear you say. Maybe we should suggest how to eliminate dandelion from the yard. Well, one way to do that is to eat it, instead of throwing the weed killer on it.

🌹 The whole plant.

🗗 Dandelion works as a diuretic, and so it may help with high blood pressure and as a weight loss aid, plus it should help normalize digestion. It is also high in iron, potassium, calcium and other minerals, plus vitamin A. The plant contains lecithin and is said to help with liver and gallbladder function.

🍽 Try nutritious dandelion greens on a salad or cooked like spinach.

☞ 2 teaspoons of root, harvested in the fall, boiled in 1 cup of water. Pick and use leaves during flowering. The juice from the stems can be used as a tonic (1 teaspoon, 3 times per day). Dandelion is also available in capsule form.

❣ Pick plants that have not been treated with herbicides and/or insecticides.

Date Palm

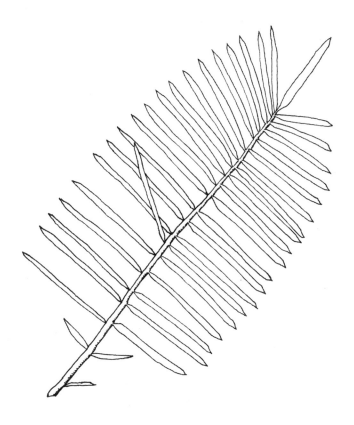

A dozen or so species of the palm that produce an edible and highly desirable fruit. A tree that is very familiar to the Bible lands and may have originated in and around old Persia, but has been cultivated in tropical and sub-tropical areas around the world. In America, date palms are most notably grown in California and Arizona. The date palm can grow to 100 feet or more, and its feathery leaves can grow to lengths of up to 20 feet. The female tree blooms white flowers and the male tree produces cream-colored flowers. The fruit develops in clusters that range from 1 to 3 inches in length and are usually dark brown, reddish- or yellow-brown, depending on the variety.

It takes two to tango, so you will need to have lots of space for planting these trees. The date palm needs full sun and a warm climate, but will grow even at seaside if the climate is an arid one. This tree can handle various types of soil as long as there is good drainage. Numerous varieties exist. Find out which one is best for your climate. The "Halawy" variety is the most cold-tolerant. The date palm can live up to and exceed 100 years!

🌹 Fruit, leaves, sap, root, and seeds.

🝚 Because the fruit is high in tannin, it may help stomach and intestinal concerns. And because the fruit is high in fiber, it makes a gentle laxative. As a tea, decoction, or syrup, dates can be used to treat sore throats, colds, and bronchial problems. The fruit has even been used to help bring down fevers, treat cystitis, edema, liver function, and even gonorrhea. A good source of vitamin A and phosphorus.

👭 Oil from the seeds is used for soap. The tree root has been used to treat toothache.

🍽 There are many uses for dates, fresh off the tree or dried. Eat whole or chop and add to cereals, breads, cakes, cookies, fruit salads, etc. Cook and eat young leaves like spinach. In India, roasted and ground date seeds are used as a coffee additive or substitute. In certain African nations, sap is tapped from the trees for making syrup.

☞ The fruit, fresh or dried, whole or chopped. Steep in water to make infusions.

📖 In the Bible, there are numerous mentions of palms and many have to do with victory and celebration. As the young nation of Israel set forth toward the Promised Land, they camped at oases where palms grew. Later, at the Feast of Tabernacles the Hebrews used palm branches to build booths to celebrate coming out of exile. At the triumphal entry of Jesus into Jerusalem, the people waved palm branches and shouted, "Hosanna, blessed is he who comes in the name of the Lord. Blessed is the King of Israel." This event was prophecy fulfilled. Jesus told the pharisees, who were there to question and criticize, that if these people did not proclaim him king, "If they keep quiet, the stones will cry out" (Lk. 19:40). On that day long ago, which we now celebrate as Palm Sunday, if the people had not proclaimed that Christ was King, God, Messiah, Savior, then creation, the very inanimate rocks themselves, would have proclaimed it. God's plan will carry on regardless of whether people acknowledge it or not! Amen!

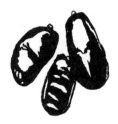

Dill

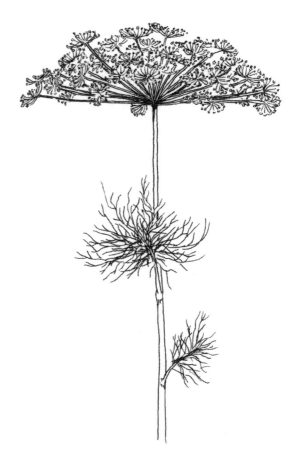

⊞ An annual plant. This is a garden favorite that you can grow among your vegetables. Stems reach 1 to 3 feet with compound umbel yellow flowers. The word dill seems to come from the words "lull" and "dull" as in the herb was used to give to restless babies to help them sleep.

☼ Easy to grow. Utilize leaves before the flower blooms. Utilize the seed at the end of the season.

❀ Flowers and leaves; also, oil is extracted.

☗ Dill is a good stomach aid for appetite promotion and upset stomach. The seed can also be chewed as a natural breath freshener.

♨ Poultices of the leaves are said to be good for treating such skin eruptions as boils and to help with reducing joint pain.

🍽 Known for years as one of the flavoring agents used in pickling cucumbers, dill is also good for cutting into fresh salads and soups. But be aware, a little goes a long way.

☞ Cut fresh leaves for salads. Use seeds for pickling of cucumbers or other vegetables.

📖 Dill has been used in the casting of spells and in witchcraft. But Jesus, in Matthew 23:23, mentions dill or anise as an offering given by the priests. Jesus chastises these hypocrites by telling them that while they may be willing to tithe a tenth of their crops, but when it comes to giving justice, mercy and faithfulness they are found lacking. The Lord's lessons are clear. Obeying the law but not showing love is not what we are to be doing. God tells us in Micah 6:8 what he wants of us, that we are to "love mercy, act justly and walk humbly with him."

❣ None noted, but dill has a strong flavor that you might find too strong if you use too much for culinary purposes.

Echinacea

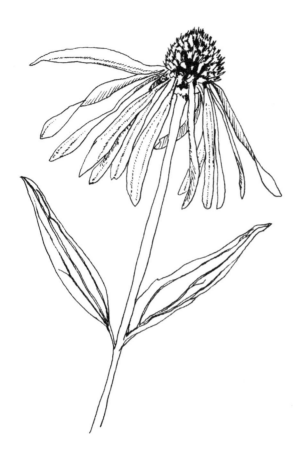

⊞ Echinacea is also known as the purple cone-flower, because of its beautiful blue, cone-shaped flower. The plant grows large and tall and has a wild look about it, but the flower is pretty and keeps its bloom for weeks. An interesting addition to the flower garden.

☼ It takes 2 years of growth for the plant to bloom. It grows tall, so plant it along fences or toward the back of the flower bed.

⚘ Rootstock.

♉ Echinacea is now considered the "wonder herb" of the decade.

Said to help the immune system fight colds, flu, and other illnesses. The jury still seems to be out on the verdict, but I have been utilizing echinacea steadily, as prescribed, for a number of years now, and have much fewer bouts with colds and flu. When I do get sick, the illness seems to be shorter and less intense. And with the controversy over antibiotic use, it is a nice alternative.

☞ Ground rootstock. I prefer to buy mine in capsules, prepared juices, or lozenges. Suggested use is in 2-week intervals, before and during the cold and flu season.

❗ People who have TB, auto-immune disease, lupus, rheumatoid arthritis, or multiple sclerosis should avoid this herb. Or check with your doctor.

Elder
(Berry)

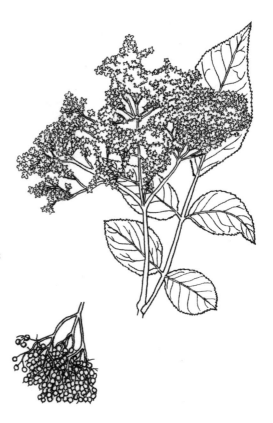

⊞ Numerous varieties include American elder, European elder, red elder and dwarf elder. Grows to 30 feet. Clusters of white or yellow flowers with a musky aroma later develop into berries. The berry stems turn a distinct red in the fall. Elderberry was once considered "the medicine chest of country people."

☼ Prefers moist, rich, well-drained soil and full to partial sun. The tree self-seeds in wild abandon, so watch out for all those suckers.

🌿 Bark, leaves, berries and flowers.

🝙 The gypsy remedy for colds and flu. A good source of vitamins A, B, and C. Considered a blood tonic, good for treating constipation and for controlling weight. The bark has been used specifically as a strong purgative, as a diuretic, and even in the treatment of epilepsy. The leaves have been used to quicken the healing of wounds. Elder flowers are said to be a good skin conditioner.

🎋 Minor skin problems such as rashes, burns, eczema. A tea of the leaves is used to spray on garden plants as an insect repellent. You can do the same for your skin. Elderberry tea rubbed on may keep away flying insects and mosquitoes.

🍽 Cooked berries are used for wine and vinegar.

☞ The bark, the leaves, the flowers and berries in teas and poultices.

📖 Steeped in lore, from Christian to the occult. Some legends suggest that this was the wood from which Christ's cross came. Others say Judas hung himself from an elderberry tree. It has been considered a symbol of death and suffering and once was grown symbolically in cemeteries. The Roman historian, Pliny, indicated that shepherds used the wood to make flutes and such. Consider the shepherds, who had seen the baby Jesus, later creating with their elder wood flutes, songs of praise for what the Lord had done.

❗ Only consume elderberries cooked, because the seeds are considered toxic. Not recommended for pregnant women.

Elecampane

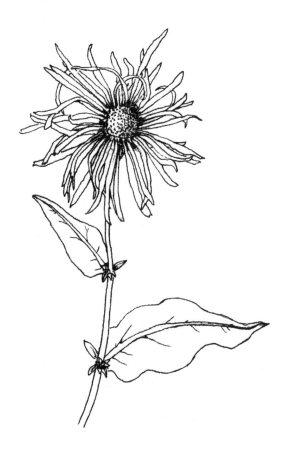

⚘ A perennial that grows to a height of 6 feet and blossoms golden-yellow flowers. The plant will remind you of a sunflower.

☼ Easy to grow; likes full to part sun and moist soil.

⚜ Rootstock; essential oil.

⛚ An herb with varied uses, such as helping to suppress coughs, improve digestion, ease urinary problems, and treat respiratory inflammations and menstrual problems. Elecampane is believed to have antibacterial and anti-fungal agents.

⋔ For the skin, specifically for scabies and itches.

☞ Utilizing the root stock in the second year of growth, use dried, powdered rootstock, 1 teaspoon per 1 cup water. Also available on the general market in syrups, lozenges, and candy, as a treatment for asthma and bronchitis.

❗ Pregnant or nursing women should check with their doctor before using elecampane.

60

Eucalyptus

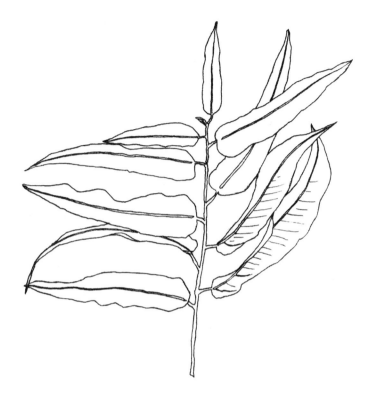

🏵 A native of Australia that grows well in the southern areas of the U.S., such as Southern California and Florida. There are many varieties. The one that is touted for its medicinal uses is the blue gum variety.

☼ Needs to grow in a warmer climate and cannot tolerate frost well. But it will grow in a pot without a great deal of care. If you can grow the tree on your property, you may find that its pungent odor chases away mosquitoes.

🌿 The leaves.

℧ A most pungent-smelling plant used as an antiseptic, deodorizer, expectorant, and stimulant. The essential oil is used for throat lozenges and other cold medicines.

👪 Used in a vapor bath or in a vaporizer for relief of congestion and asthma. Said to be good for treating minor wounds. Naturally-made deodorants often contain eucalyptus.

☞ Utilize leaves for vapor. Utilize oil for internal purposes, such as throat lozenges, or for external purposes, such as a salve for stiff joints and sore muscles.

❗ This is a very strong herb that should only be used in moderation—probably not internally, except as a throat lozenge. Can irritate already-sensitive skin.

Evening Primrose

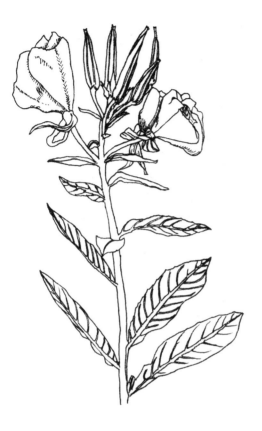

⊞ A biennial or annual plant, depending upon climate. Some varieties grow large, to 6 feet with 6-inch leaves. Blooms pink or yellow lemon-scented flowers, up to 2½ inches long, from early summer to late fall, depending on variety. The name evening primrose comes from the fact that some varieties bloom in the late afternoon and evening hours.

☼ Easy to grow, but invasive. Evening primrose makes a good ground cover in difficult-to-grow areas.

🌺 The whole plant.

🗲 As a tea or oil it is used to control coughing associated with colds, or for asthma. It has been recommended for mild depression. Said to be helpful in proper function of the liver, spleen, and digestive system. Evening primrose has high amounts of gamma linolenic acid, which is good for many body functions. The oil may lower cholesterol and high blood pressure conditions. In recent times, evening primrose has become highly touted for the relief it provides women suffering the symptoms of PMS.

👪 Used as an ointment for rashes and skin irritations. It may help with eczema and give you more healthy-looking skin. Often used for babies with "cradle cap."

🍴 All parts are edible and the rootstock is said to taste similar to parsnip.

☞ Use the plant (1 teaspoon herb per 1 cup water), the oil, or capsule form.

❗ Don't use evening primrose if you suffer from migraines or epilepsy.

Eyebright

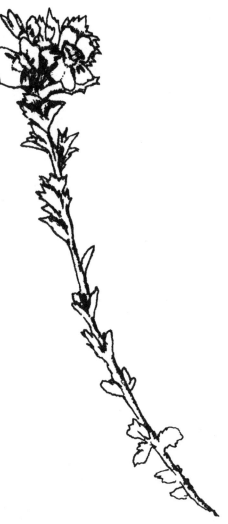

🏵 A small plant with a downy appearance that grows only to a maximum of 12 inches. White flowers that are decorated with splashes of red, purple, or yellow bloom early summer to early fall. Past writers describing the flower have suggested that it looks like a blood-shot eye!

☼ No tips on how to grow. Eyebright grows as a wild-flower in meadows and pastures. It's difficult to cultivate because it needs grasses to grow in.

🌿 Predominantly the flower when it is in full bloom in the height of summer. It is the fluid or oil from the flower that is used medicinally.

🝔 The name tells it all as for its main use, and that is in treating eye inflammations, eye strains, and other eye-related concerns. Use of this herb may help with eye problems related to colds and allergies.

👬 Used as an eyewash to relieve the above-mentioned symptoms.

☞ One suggestion is to make a weak tea to directly wash into the eyes. Use 1 teaspoon per 1 cup water. Eyebright is also available commercially as an oil or in capsule form.

❗ None noted, but before directly applying to your eyes, check with your doctor or herbalist.

Fennel
(Sweet)

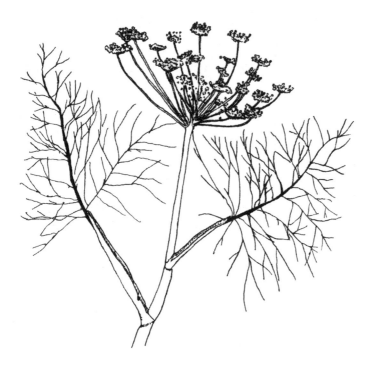

✿ A biennial or perennial plant, depending upon climate, fennel was transplanted from the Bible lands, and now is found growing wild in North America. It grows a long carrot-type root, long stems, and large umbels of yellow flowers from summer to early fall. The plant can grow 3 to 5 feet, and is similar to dill.

☼ Easy to grow, drought resistant. Fennel adds a wild and unique look to the traditional garden.

🌿 Root, seeds, and leaves.

☕ The seeds and root are used for a variety of stomach concerns from gas and cramps to colic. Fennel may also be used in gargles for coughs and a raspy sore throat. It is also said to stimulate the production of mother's milk.

🏵 Fennel oil can be used to give relief to joints inflamed by arthritis and rheumatism. A decoction of the seeds can be used as an eye wash.

🍽 Found in most spice shelves, fennel seeds are used in fish dishes, soups, stews, and sauces. The tender young stalks are served in salads or sautéed with a little garlic and olive oil. Note a surprising, mild licorice flavor. And if you don't like the seeds, the birds will be glad to eat them.

☞ If you are going to extract oil from fennel root, gather in the spring of the plant's second year. Use the seeds, 1 teaspoonful to 1 cup water as a tea for internal use. As an eyewash, use ½ teaspoon per 1 cup water. Combine a few drops of oil with 1 tablespoon honey for coughs and sore throats.

📖 Fennel is related to caraway and dill, which are mentioned in the Bible.

Fenugreek

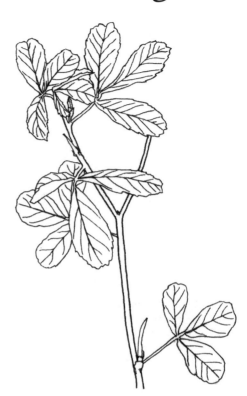

⌘ Grown as an annual, this plant is cultivated for its seeds. Fenugreek basically means, "Greek hay" because it was used as animal fodder. Plant grows to 2 feet tall with a long tap root. The leaves are triangular in shape, the flower a pale yellow, and the plant is considered a legume because of the pod that contains 16-20 seeds.

✿ Grow it as you would peas, in well drained and fertile soil with lots of available sun. This is an easy plant to grow although not particularly attractive.

✿ Seeds, pulverized in teas or poultices. Also available in capsule form. Although the seeds taste bitter, oil of fenugreek is said to have a slight maple flavor.

☡ The use of this herb can be dated back to the time of the ancient Assyrians and the Egyptian pharaohs. They, as have countless generations of people, used it to help relieve symptoms of sore throats and the respiratory complaints of colds and bronchitis. However, there is much more to this herb. This herb qualifies as a whole-body tonic and cleanser. Fenugreek can help reduce fevers and lower cholesterol and blood sugars. Earl Mindell indicates that research has been done on fenugreek and the possible help it gives with the control of diabetes. There is suggestion that it is good for the eyes, may help with milk production for lactating mothers and for symptoms of menopause.

🏛 Seeds made into a paste may help with skin irritations, the discomfort of swollen glands, and even fibromyalgia.

🍽 The fresh leaves and dried seeds have been used for culinary purposes for millenniums. The plant is high in vitamins and minerals, so it may be an interesting alternative to spinach.

☞ The fresh leaves for culinary uses. The seeds pulverized for internal and external medicinal uses.

📖 None noted, but this is an ancient herb that would have been known by the people of the Bible times.

Feverfew

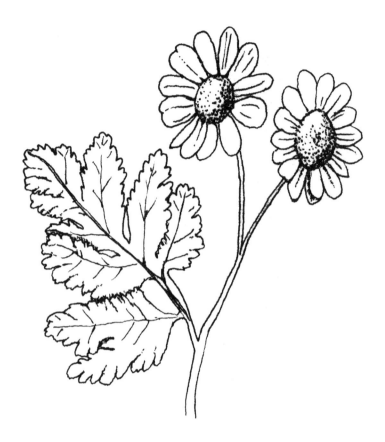

✿ A perennial that is part of the chrysanthemum family. It grows to 2 feet tall, with lots of small daisy-like, white-and-yellow flowers that bloom from late spring into fall.

☼ A pretty plant in the garden; but you'd best keep it in a pot or a contained area, because the intrusive plant spreads rapidly.

🌿 The whole plant.

☕ As its name suggests, feverfew was used before the days of aspirin, to reduce fever. It lost favor for a long time, but has been rediscovered in this new season of herbal awareness for treating the symptoms and related problems of migraines.

☞ 1 teaspoon plant parts with 1 cup water, or use capsule form.

❗ A powerful herb that may cause ulcers of the mouth. If you are pregnant, it is suggested that you avoid feverfew. Check with a respected herbalist before using.

Fig

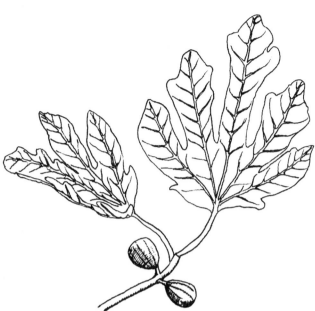

A deciduous tree native to the Mediterranean, fig is now cultivated in many places in the world. The tree can reach heights of 30 feet. Bark is heavy, smooth, gray-colored; leaves have 3 to 5 lobes. The flower is found inside the fruit—that is why, when you open a fig you will notice that the interior has a flower-like appearance. In some species, pollination takes place when certain insects enter the fruit. The ripe fig is greenish yellow, brown, or purple, depending upon variety, of which there are many.

☼ More commonly grown in sub-tropical and tropical areas, I have seen fig cultivated as far north as Vancouver, Washington, against the sunny, south side of structures. The ripe fruit of those trees was very tasty. You can grow a fig tree in a large pot or tub, taking it inside during the winter. It will grow in average soil, but needs much sun and good drainage. Drought resistant.

The fruit.

Considered a good and safe laxative, fig is high in fiber. Try fig when you have a cold, as it is said to help treat the mucous membranes.

Herbal authority John Lust suggests cutting a fig in half and applying it directly to a boil. He must be on the right track, because the prophet Isaiah suggested that fig be made into a poultice to treat a boil on King Hezekiah (Isa. 38:21). Also, the stems and leaves are pressed for juice to remove warts.

Because they are good fresh or dried, you can find many uses for the fruit. In the Old Testament, Abigail made fig into cakes. I like dried figs, dates, and raisins in oatmeal, or even better, in oatmeal cookies with honey used as a sweetener!

Numerous. The first clothes worn by Adam and Eve were fig leaves. The evil Syrian king, Sennacherib, promised the nation of Israel that everyone would have their own fig tree if they'd surrender to him. God had different plans; the angel of the Lord wiped out the king's huge army while they slept. Later, the loss of figs and other staples was caused by sin and punishment when God called the people to repentance: "It is because they have forsaken my law, which I set before them" (Jer. 9:13).

67

Flax

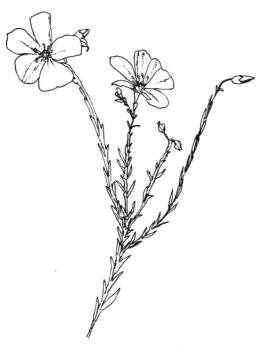

🌸 An annual or perennial, depending on climate, flax is a sun-loving plant that grows up to 3 feet tall with unique 5-petal, violet-blue flowers that bloom only for a day. But the plant continues to produce blooms through the heat of the summer. The fruit or seed grows in pods of 8 to 10 seeds.

☼ Easy to grow; drought-resistant; good for areas where it is difficult to grow flowers.

🌹 The mature seeds.

🍵 Much study has been done on the dietary benefits of flax seed. High in alpha-linoleic acid, flax is believed to fight cancer and protect the stomach and colon. The seeds are used to relieve cough and congestion, aid digestion, and combat constipation. Flax is said to help with urinary problems. It may help keep high blood pressure down, aid in developing strong bones, teeth and nails, and help in the fight against osteoporosis. You may also make tea or purchase cold-pressed oil.

👥 Use in a similar manner to fennel, for treating rheumatism. Boil 1 teaspoon flax seed in 1 quart water until ½ quart is left. Apply as a hot compress in a linen wrap to affected areas.

🍽 Add the oil, seeds, or meal to breads, breakfast cereals, etc.

📖 When the two Hebrews came to spy out the Promised Land, Rahab hid them on her roof under the flax she had gathered there to dry. Because she chose to protect the spies, at risk to her own safety, they promised that if she would hang a scarlet cord (probably made of flax) out her window, they'd spare her and her family when they attacked Jericho. (See Josh. 2) Early Christians considered this blood-colored cord a symbol of Christ's atonement. Rahab became part of God's great cloud of witnesses mentioned in Hebrews Chapter 11.

Flax reeds were bruised and beaten to make cloth and wicks. Isaiah prophesied, "A bruised reed he will not break, and a smoldering wick he will not snuff out" (Isa. 42:3). Jesus comes to mend broken lives. Then, like the wick of an oil lamp, you can let your light shine. Because of Christ, you may shine like a lamp in a dark place and like stars in the universe "as you hold out the Word of life" (see Phil. 2:15-16).

❗ The immature seeds are considered poisonous. If using flax as a laxative, drink plenty of water.

Frankincense

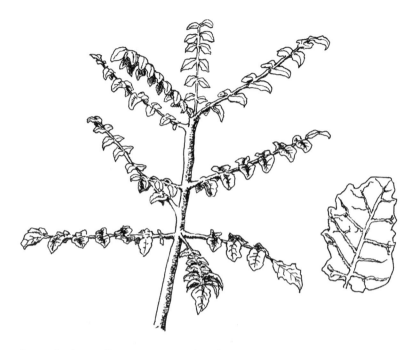

⊕ Resin from the boswellia tree, a most familiar plant in Bible times.

🜲 The bark is utilized in oils, perfumes, and incense.

☞ This substance is rare and expensive. I mainly use it as an anointing oil in healing services, applying anointing oil to a person seeking healing.

📖 Mentioned at least fourteen times in the Bible. Leviticus 2:2 mentions it as a substance to be used as a burnt offering and an aroma pleasing to the Lord. King Solomon and his entourage were compared to the burning smoke of incense. Frankincense and royalty go hand in hand.

The three magi brought the baby Jesus gifts of gold, frankincense, and myrrh. Jesus came to be "God with us." Frankincense reminds us that a unique and unprecedented thing took place when Jesus was born. God came to be with his creation. While remaining God, he became a man—God sharing our existence with us.

I think of frankincense as an herb of prayer. In Revelation, where we are given incredible visions of the final conflict and of our future heavenly home, we read that "four living creatures and the twenty-four elders fell down before the Lamb... holding golden bowls full of incense, which are the prayers of the saints" (Rev. 5:8). Think about this for a moment, and then rejoice! To God our prayers are fine incense held in golden bowls. When you struggle in prayer and think that what you bring before the Lord is unimportant, let this beautiful description help you see how God feels about your prayers. Then "in everything, by prayer and petition, with thanksgiving, present your requests to God" (Phil. 4:6).

Garlic

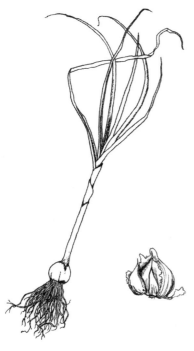

⚜ The common garlic of which there are numerous varieties, including the favorite elephant garlic. Considered a wonder herb in these modern days; it was also very popular in Bible times.

✿ Garlic grows easily and in many climates, year round. Consider planting garlic around areas where moles are active, and you may find that they will leave. Also plant in around herbs and vegetables that are more susceptible to insects, and it may help keep the pests away. Just the right amount of water is needed. Use too much and you get lots of stalk, use too little and you get small heads. I'm still learning this lesson but my latest crop was the best yet, so keep experimenting. If you have figured out how to grow large onions, then grow the garlic in a similar fashion. However, keep in mind, garlic grows at a slower rate.

🌿 The bulb, cloves and seeds.

🗡 Garlic has long been known as a cure-all for the entire digestive system, but it also regulates the gall bladder and the liver. From Louis Pasteur to Dr. Albert Schweitzer many have discovered that garlic kills dangerous microorganisms and can be used to treat cholera, typhoid, and dysentery. It's also found to be helpful for the heart and circulation and is beneficial for proper blood pressure. It will help to lower the bad cholesterol and raise the levels of the beneficial one. There is even a suggestion that garlic can destroy some types of cancer cells.

� Oil of the garlic can be used for earaches, sprains, muscle aches and skin disorders. Of course the more you use it, the more people will know you use it.

🍽 Nearly endless; so, knowing all that you now know, experiment.

☞ Make a tea from some chopped garlic cloves in a quart of water. There are also odorless capsules available if you don't like the smell.

📖 Historical accounts indicate that slaves in Egypt were given garlic to strengthen them for building pyramids. We know that the Hebrews were held captive and forced to work for the Egyptians. They prospered in health and numbers in slavery, so the garlic must have helped. Garlic is only mentioned once, in Numbers 11:5, as the Hebrews complained about what they had lost. And God was providing them manna from heaven! But people will complain about anything. For some self-centered people, God himself won't satisfy. "Taste and see that the Lord is good" (Ps. 34:8).

❗ One word of caution: garlic is a strong herb, so too much consumption could cause an allergic reaction.

70

Ginger

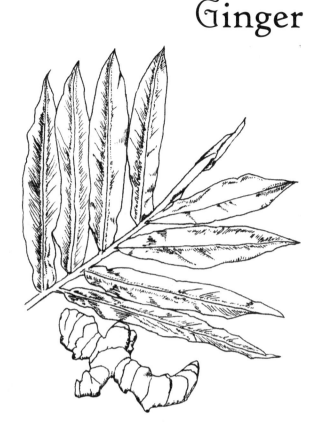

▦ This perennial plant grows an aromatic, thick root. The plant has one simple, leafy stem 3 or 4 feet long. The flower is white with violet streaks. This long-time favorite of tropical Asia is enjoying a comeback worldwide because of its varied health benefits.

☼ In America, ginger is cultivated in the south from Florida to southern California, and Hawaii. To grow your own, plant it in raised beds so to promote proper root growth. In harsher climates, you can grow ginger in a greenhouse.

🌿 The root.

♆ Your first thought of ginger might be your grandmother's gingersnap cookies. I can also remember my mother giving me ginger ale when I had the stomach flu as a way to bring relief to my troubled tummy. My wife bakes wonderful gingersnaps and I can't get enough of them. They taste great, and they are soothing to the digestive system. It is also considered to be one of the few safe substances to help pregnant women deal with morning sickness. If you have a tendency to get "car sick," "air sick," or "sea sick," a little ginger may help your symptoms. There seems to be evidence that ginger can reduce cholesterol levels, lower blood pressure, and ward off blood clots that could trigger heart attacks.

♜ Mixed with olive oil, it may be good as a natural remedy to relieve dandruff or soothe an earache.

🍽 A requirement in many Asian foods, ginger can also be used in a number of recipes. Try it in cooked carrots you will double your herbal benefits. Try it in anything, and see what you think.

☞ Grate fresh ginger for teas, compresses, and culinary purposes. Also available in capsules.

📖 Ginger is known to have long been used in the lands of the Bible. It was thought to help with leprosy. The Hebrew people would have used it as a regular part of their diet, trading or purchasing the herb from traveling spice dealers.

Ginkgo

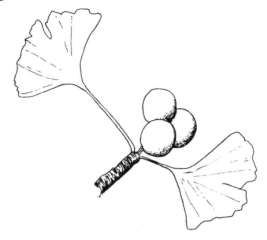

🏵 This is one of my favorite herbs because of its benefits and because of its unique appearance. An ancient tree, probably present in the Garden of Eden, ginkgo became nearly extinct until it was saved a century ago. The ginkgo tree averages a height of about 50 feet, but can grow to 80 feet. It has fan-shaped, leathery leaves. For harsh climates or for small areas, you can confine the tree to a pot. Some people have even turned the tree into a bonsai.

✿ Best to plant male trees, because the fruit of the female tree is messy and smelly. The tree likes sun and a good soil. Stake the tree in the first years of life and water through dry seasons until it reaches over 10 feet tall.

🌿 The leaves.

🗘 Ginkgo is considered one of the miracle herbs of the last century because of its many uses and benefits for the stressed-out generations of these modern times. Much research is being done on this herb. It is said to help improve circulation, improve mental functioning, and may relieve symptoms of Alzheimer's disease and the effects of stroke. It also seems to help with vertigo and tinnitus (ringing in the ears). This is because it seems to increase blood flow to the brain and the lower extremities. I notice that if I take it on a regular basis, the nearly constant ringing in my ears is lessened, and sometimes even eliminated. I have hearing loss from the damage caused by rupturing my eardrums in the military. As I grow older, it seems my hearing lessens and the tinnitus increases. Ginkgo is the only thing I've found that combats this aggravating condition. Ginkgo may make the aging process a little easier by slowing down the loss of function. It may help prevent cancer, because it is full of antioxidants. Ginkgo even helps in the treatment of hemorrhoids.

☞ Use leaf and oil extract for teas. Also available in capsule form. Now added to juices, natural sodas, and other items. I drink a product called "Intellijuice" produced by the Hansen's Beverage Co. I don't know whether it makes me any more intelligent; but it sure gives me a mental lift.

❗ Avoid ginkgo at night if you are hoping for a good night's sleep.

Ginseng

American   Chinese   Siberian

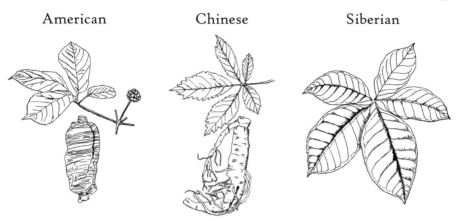

▣ A favorite, with many benefits. Considered to be a "wonder herb." All are perennials. The Chinese has an aromatic root that grows to 2 feet, blooms a single-umbel, green-to-yellow flower early in summer. The American species is similar in appearance, but the root splits into a fork. "Ginseng" derived from the expression "root of man" because the root grows in the shape of the human body. Ginseng is one of the oldest, continuously-used herbs. Siberian ginseng is not closely related to the others, but is similar in appearance.

✿ American ginseng prefers cool climate and rich soil. Found in woodlands, it's the most available for garden use. But it's difficult to grow, and usually doesn't mature for use until 6 to 9 years.

✿ The root.

🍶 All have similar uses, but many authorities say the potency is strongest in the Chinese variety, which is utilized for the control of blood sugar levels, blood pressure, and circulation. Many consider it a blood tonic. It has a stimulating effect and is a good alternative to caffeine because, unlike caffeine, it won't let you down quickly. It helps the body deal with stress. Women use it to control hot flashes and other symptoms of menopause. It may also help in the control of cholesterol. Long before these attributes were discovered, ginseng was (and still is) considered an aphrodisiac. It energizes and seems to increase overall physical stamina. American ginseng seems to be less powerful, but is helpful in relieving a queasy stomach. Siberian ginseng is a recognized cure for insomnia, and it is said to help with bronchitis and other ailments of the lungs.

🍽 None noted, but I have found ginseng cola is a nice alternative to colas that are full of caffeine, sugar or sugar substitutes, and other harmful chemicals. Try one in the early afternoon, or after heavy exertion.

☞ The root stalk is dried and ground and made into capsules, extract, and oils.

❗ Seems to be very safe when taken responsibly. But avoid use of Chinese and American ginseng at bedtime, or you may find yourself awake all night.

Goldenseal

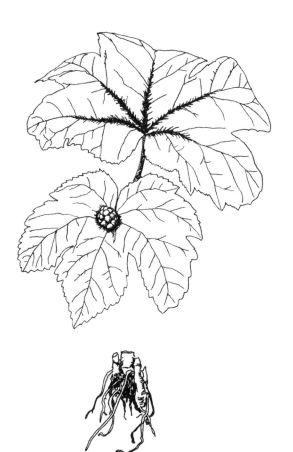

⚜ A small perennial plant, native to North America and found in eastern areas. One stem grows to a foot, topped by a single flower of greenish white. Goldenseal has been called by some the "poor man's ginseng." It's a multipurpose herb with a number of benefits.

☼ Like ginseng, goldenseal is difficult to grow. It needs more shade than sun. The soil should be a rich compost material similar to what you would find on a forest floor. It will take 2 to 3 years for the plant to develop a harvestable root.

🌱 The root.

☕ Goldenseal acts as a stomach aid and laxative.

It seems to have good effect on the mucous membranes and is used to treat cold and flu symptoms. Many feel it is best used for treating symptoms of stress, anxiety, nervousness, and exhaustion.

👪 Women have used it for treating vaginal infections. It has been used to treat skin disorders, ringworm, as an eye wash, and even for treating STDs.

☞ Capsules, ground root stock, and extract are all available and it is best to utilize it per instructions from your herbalist, because this is a powerful herb with some cautionary concerns.

📖 None noted. Jesuit priests in early North America used it to treat cuts and wounds.

❗ This is a powerful herb that should not be taken by pregnant women or by people with high blood pressure. Taking goldenseal has a cumulative effect, so proper dosage is very important. Do not take it longer than 2 weeks at a time. And beware that the fresh plant could be poisonous to eat.

Gotu Kola

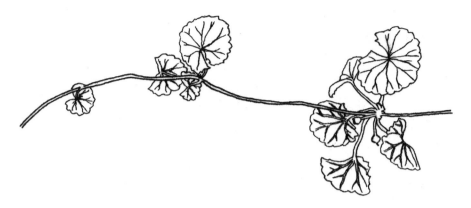

🏵 When you first see the name you are inclined to wonder if this herb has anything to do with the cola nut and the cola beverages that we in America are so fond of. That isn't it. But this is an herb whose use goes back to ancient times in India and then later in China. Called, by some, the "smartweed," this plant grows in the tropical regions. It hugs the ground with bright shiny leaves, up to 2 inches in size, growing in a trailing pattern. A few red flowers bloom beneath the leaves. Gotu kola is originally native to East Asia, but has been introduced to the tropical climates of Hawaii and Mexico where it is considered a weed. It is now also found in the southern portions of the U.S., growing in low elevation wetlands.

☼ The plant can be cultivated indoors.

🌱 Nuts, roots and seeds.

☡ Gotu kola is considered a tonic for frazzled nerves, but it is also said to be effective in treating colds and upper respiratory complaints and even bowel problems. Much study has been done on this herb because of its positive effect upon the circulatory system. Many people take it as a blood tonic, and it may help with leg cramps and the potentially-serious condition of phlebitis. Because gotu kola is effective on the circulation, it may give help similar to that of ginkgo in improving memory and brain function. It's considered "brain food" by many. This herb seems to be effective for women's reproductive health in the speeding of healing after women have had episiotomies during childbirth. It may also be a natural remedy for decreased sex drive in both men and women. The herb has even been used to treat leprosy.

☞ The nuts, roots, and seeds are usually dried and turned into powder for tinctures and capsules.

❣ Utilizing large amounts can have a narcotic effect and can cause headaches, vertigo, and even comas. If you are pregnant, check with your doctor because there may be some concerns. And if you have thyroid problems, you should check with your doctor before taking gotu kola. This is a powerful herb that should be used only as directed.

Grape

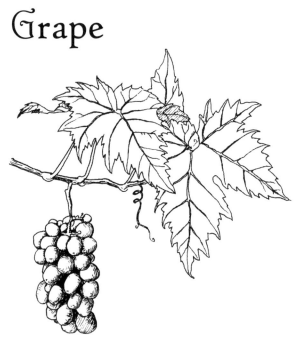

⊛ A deciduous vine grown throughout the world and in many climates, that produces an abundance of fruit formed in bunches.

☼ A fast-growing plant that can easily double its size in a year. There are two basic types of grape: those used for wine, and those used for general table consumption. Find a variety that fits your climate. For ornamental appearance, grow on an arbor or fence. Vines growing over wood fences create a cool patio cover in sunny, hot places.

🌿 The whole fruit; extracts of skin and seed.

📇 High in fiber. Contains: high amounts of boron, which may help in the fight against osteoporosis; tannins, which may help fight off viruses; vitamins A, B, and C, calcium, potassium, and zinc, which may strengthen the immune system. Clark Hansen, a doctor of naturopathic medicine, indicates grape seed contains high amounts of procyanidolic oligomers which he believes are 20 times more potent than vitamin C and 50 times more potent than vitamin E as an antioxidant. He has found grape seed extract, in his own practice, helpful in treating or preventing arthritis, allergies, hardening of the arteries, ulcers, skin wrinkles, cellulite, liver spots, hemorrhoids, varicose veins, gum disease, cancer, strokes, cataracts, glaucoma and diabetes.

👪 Grape juice is said to help fight tooth decay.

🍽 Many. For one thing, I add an array of fresh herbs to red wine vinegar, let it sit a couple weeks, then use it in preparing many foods.

☞ Much study has been done on using the skin and the seed extracts, plus the value of the vinegar. I think the best way to enjoy grape is to eat the fruit fresh by the bunch. As studies continue, many new benefits will probably be discovered.

📖 Grapes grow well in the Bible lands. They're first mentioned when Noah planted a vineyard. But his wine consumption became his undoing (Gen. 9). Later, the men Moses sent to explore the land of Canaan cut one branch of grapes from a vine and had to carry it on a pole between them because the grape clusters were so heavy (Num. 13). Vineyards were valued highly and watchtowers were built to protect the vines from animals and thieves. In one of Jesus' most appealing parables, he refers to himself as the grapevine, to believers as the branches, and to the Father as the gardener.

Hawthorn

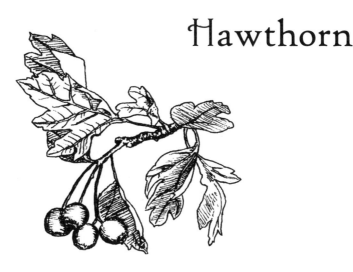

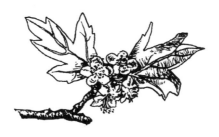

⊞ A tree or shrub that originated in Europe. Distinctive, with thorny branches, shiny leaves, and white flowers that bloom late spring and early summer, developing red berries in the fall.

✿ The tree can grow to 25 feet in most climates.

🌿 The flowers, but specifically the berries.

⛏ Hawthorn is another herb that is one of my favorites and one that has been embraced lately as an herb that acts as a heart tonic. I have found for myself that it helps keep the blood pressure down. There is much study being done on this plant, because of the possibility that it helps to strengthen weakened heart muscle. Said to be good for nervousness and insomnia.

🍽 Hawthorn is used in many herbal teas.

☞ Use 1 teaspoon crushed flowers per 1 cup water; or add 1 cup boiling water to 2 teaspoons of berries. Also available in capsule form.

📖 This tree produces an abundance of berries which birds eat to help them get through the winter. But the tree is also covered with thorns. It reminds me that Jesus wore a crown of thorns and put up with much abuse on my behalf, to give me life.

Horehound

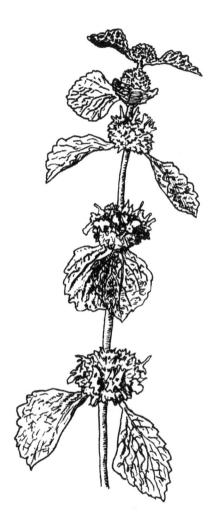

⚙ If you have been around for many years, then this is a familiar herb. In days past, horehound candy and throat lozenges were regular items in the candy stores and at the pharmacy. Horehound is related to the mint family and is a very unique and unusual-looking plant with its wrinkly leaves, thick squarish stem, and small white flowers. A perennial, it grows like an annual in harsher climates.

☼ Horehound is an interesting addition to the garden. It grows fairly well in a pot or in your garden with no special treatment. You can propagate it from roots, cuttings, or seed.

❀ The whole plant.

✇ Horehound is enjoying a new popularity. While in Vermont, I bought horehound candy; and it tasted very good, and was soothing to the throat. Horehound is also a stomach aid. On a hot summer day, when you are feeling sluggish and over-heated, use it as one of your ingredients for a summer iced tea, because it has a cooling effect upon the body.

⸙ Horehound is a good topical treatment for persistent skin problems. The tea or crushed leaves can be applied to skin rashes, itches, and to promote the healing of wounds.

🍽 None noted, except for candy and cough lozenges; but you can sprinkle the leaves on a salad.

☞ Steep 1 teaspoon herb in ½ cup boiling water.

📖 Known as a bitter herb, horehound can be used in Passover celebrations.

Horseradish

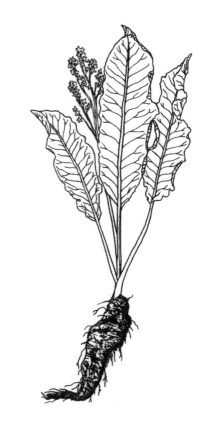

⬡ Perennial. Keeps coming back year after year, whether you want it to or not. Grows 3 feet of leaves above ground and a tap root with many offshoots up to 3 feet underground. This sun lover can handle a dry climate. Growing and processing this plant can be a heady experience. I grew some one year, dug up the roots and took them inside to grind in the food processor. The grinding activated fumes that invaded our eyes and nasal cavities and literally drove us out of the house, and the whole neighborhood smelled of fresh horseradish.

✿ Very intrusive. I planted it at the corner of a raised garden box. It sent out shoots underground and grew so big, it separated the corners of the box.

🌿 The root.

⛉ As a digestive aid, a diuretic, and to aid in the breakup of congestion and mucus from respiratory cold symptoms. Mixed with honey, it is said to help get rid of a stubborn cough.

👭 Used (carefully) as a topical in the treatment of rheumatism. Use ground horseradish mixed with cornstarch wrapped in a bandage and applied directly to the afflicted area. Avoid direct contact with sensitive skin areas.

🍴 Excellent with meats, it adds flavor and helps to assimilate the meat quicker through the digestive system, which is good because meats can be slow movers.

☞ Finely ground, turned into a paste, often adding oil, vinegar, mayonnaise and such. The original Passover eaters may have taken in an undiluted dose that really would have reminded them of the tears they and their ancestors shed while in bondage and slavery to the Egyptian pharaohs.

📖 Very familiar to the people of the Bible lands where it both grew wild and was cultivated. It's most notably related to the Passover. The strong flavor and fumes provide strong symbolism to the Jewish and Christian faiths.

❗ A very strong herb. Can burn the skin. Over-use can cause diarrhea and profuse, excessive sweating. One time my wife and I were out with friends for steak dinner in a dimly lit room. On my wife's plate the horseradish sat next to the mashed potatoes. With her mind on the conversation, Kit scooped up a forkful of horseradish. It burned so badly, she saw stars and literally couldn't talk for minutes. A little goes a long way! One plant will probably provide more root for your use than you will ever need.

Hyssop

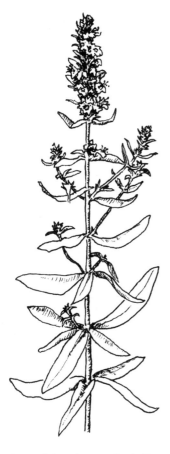

⚘ Another great favorite of mine that has spiritual significance, this pretty plant is considered an evergreen. It has nice blue flowers that blossom the whole of summer, and they will look good in your flower bed. If you live in a northern climate, this plant will only last as an annual.

☼ Grows easily. Likes sun. Young plants require more water.

🌿 The entire plant.

♉ Hyssop is a great all-around herb touted to be powerful enough to have anti-viral properties.

👫 As astringent, used topically. Also a gargle for sore throats, coughs, colds.

🍽 Utilize it like mint, and see what you think.

📖 Mentioned many times in the Bible, hyssop was used as a brush to paint the door frames with blood to keep away the angel of death during the days of Moses. For 400 years the Hebrews suffered under slavery in Egypt, until God set them free and sent them to the Promised Land.

One of the plagues God directed towards Egypt, when Pharaoh would not let the slaves go, brought death to every first-born boy child of both the Egyptians and the Jews. God instructed Moses to tell the Jews to take hyssop and paint their door frames with lamb's blood. When the angel of death came by and saw the blood, he would pass over that household. The long, bushy hyssop plant would be dipped in the lamb's blood, then wiped first left to right and then up and down, painting the sign of a cross. From very early days, God made people aware of the cross and the cost that he would pay to deliver his people from the slavery of sin.

Hyssop has astringent, cleansing properties. "Cleanse me with hyssop, and I will be clean; wash me, and I will be whiter than snow" (Ps. 51:7). It was used in priestly ceremonies in seeking forgiveness for the people.

On a hyssop branch, gall was offered to Jesus on the cross for relief of pain. But he refused it. The sinless one took the anguish and the dirt of our sins upon himself so that we could be cleansed from our sin.

❗ A strong herb. Don't use for extended periods unless your doctor advises it.

Iceland Moss

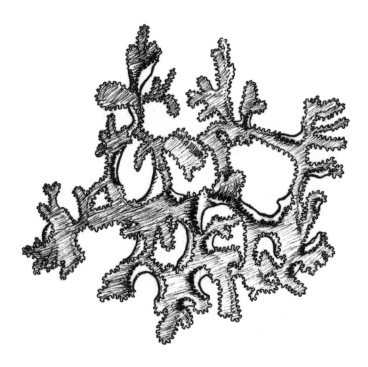

⚘ Iceland moss is not a moss at all, but a lichen. This is a common plant found in many Northern countries in cool, damp areas. The little plant grows no taller than a few inches and may appear in colors of green to gray, sometimes flecked with red.

☼ None noted. Gather this herb in the wild places.

⚘ The whole plant.

▯ Iceland moss has antiseptic qualities and is a tonic for the mucous membranes. Iceland moss is helpful for chronic pulmonary problems such as chest colds and bronchitis, and has even been touted for use in the treatment of tuberculosis. Iceland moss helps with digestive disturbances and dysentery problems. For nursing mothers the lichen may be helpful in milk production, but as with anything, check with your doctor or naturopath.

🍽 *Peterson Field Guides: Edible Wild Plants* indicates that this plant can be used to make a flour or added to a soup. The plant must be cooked for a long time, however, to make it palatable.

☞ The tradition is to gather the plant in the dry weather of late spring to late summer. Grind into a powder and then drink in a decoction.

❗ Large amounts or extended use can cause stomach problems.

Jasmine

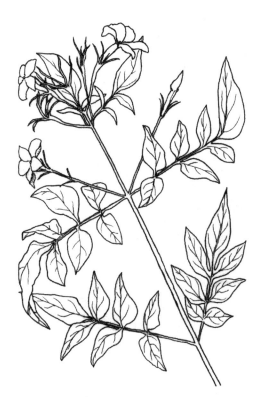

⚜ Specifically, white jasmine (*Jasminum officinale*) although well over 100 varieties exist throughout the world. The British brought it to Europe, climatized the plant so many of us in Northern populations can enjoy this fragrant climbing vine. The leaves are small and a darker green, and a multitude of white blossoms bloom June to October.

☼ Grows in most climates of the U.S. and winters over in fairly harsh climates. The plant will grow from 12 to 20 feet but requires support. Mine grow over an arbor at a gate. The plant should be allowed to grow and flourish until fall, then as the flowers die off and the plant moves into winter mode, it should be pruned substantially for prolific growth next spring.

🌿 Specifically the flower. I included this herb because of the aromatherapy it provides just being near it and the highly favorable and fragrant jasmine tea that made a comeback in the 1960s. In India, jasmine is used to treat snakebite and the leaves are used to treat the eye.

🛡 As a tea to calm the senses and help regulate the digestive system, and for the treatment of mild respiratory problems brought on by colds, etc.

⚕ The oil for use as a skin tonic.

🍽 Utilize the flowers to brighten up and flavor other teas.

☞ Fresh flowers steeped in hot water for a tea.

📖 None specifically, but in old religious paintings you may notice jasmine plants painted into pictures that depict the Virgin Mary. Maybe the sweetness of the flower reminded the artists of the sweetness of the greatest woman who ever lived and who was considered highly esteemed by God. As announced by the Angel Gabriel, "Greetings, you who are highly favored! The Lord is with you" (Lk. 1:28).

❢ Other parts of the plant are considered potentially poisonous, and in some varieties the entire plant is considered poisonous.

Juniper

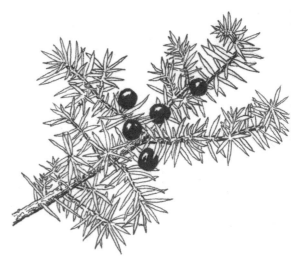

❁ *Juniperus communis* and *Juniperus oxycedrus*. I've spent much of my life near these unique trees, evergreens with prickly grayish-green leaves and gray-brown rough bark. Related to the cedar. Most varieties not large, but shrubby. Highly aromatic. Slow growing. Junipers bear bluish-black berries that take two years to develop. Old weather prognosticators predict how heavy the winter snows will be by the amount of berries the tree produces. Eaten in abundance by birds and animals.

☼ Found wild in the west. Unlikely you'd want to add to the abundance unless you live where they don't grow and want one as an ornamental. An arid to semi-arid plant; too much water, humidity, and too little sun will kill it.

� The dried berries.

☞ As a diuretic, helpful for urinary tract complaints and as Earl Mindell points out, "successful in treating gout." Berries have also been used as a digestive aid and for the easing of abdominal cramps.

👫 Utilize the oil to be rubbed into joints specifically for gouty conditions. The vapors of the oil in a bath or a humidifier are said to help with congestion from colds and bronchial problems. The oil is also used in cosmetics and perfumes.

🍽 Flavor is similar to rosemary. Try a few crushed juniper berries on veal or lamb.

☞ The fresh or dried berries and the extracted oil. The berries are crushed and steeped in hot water. The berries should be dried before being consumed.

📖 Juniper in Europe and the Middle East was called "broom tree," to which there are references in the Bible. I like 1 Kings 19:3-9. The great prophet Elijah was running at low ebb and was tired. "He came to a broom tree, sat down under it and prayed that he might die. 'I have had enough, Lord,' he said, 'Take my life'." Sometimes we've just had enough! And we're ready for the Lord to take us home. But God wasn't done with Elijah. After a few naps under the shade of the juniper, plus nourishment provided on the wings of angels, Elijah was strengthened to carry on. The next time I am weary from a desert hike and rest in the shade of an old gnarly juniper, I'll think about how God strengthens us when we think, "Lord, I've had enough." Elijah received God's strengthening and protection, then went on to fulfill God's purpose for him.

❗ This is a strong herb. Pregnant women should avoid it because it's said to stimulate the uterus. People with kidney disease should avoid using juniper.

Kava Kava

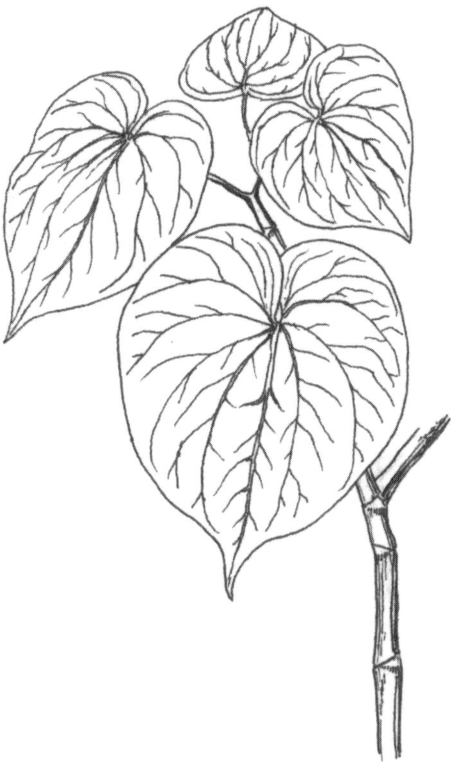

I've included kava kava (*Piper methysticum*) because of its current popularity. This is a tropical plant of the South Seas Islands also cultivated in Australia and the U.S. Kava kava has been in use for centuries, but in recent decades has become very popular in America. This plant was discovered by Europeans because of the great ocean explorer James Cook. He may have given it the nickname, "intoxicating pepper." Kava kava is a flowering shrub, with wide oblong leaves, that grows only a few feet tall. It is the rhizome or root, similar to ginger, that is used. Natives fermented the root and used it for religious purposes. The chewing of the root has an intoxicating effect. This method of use is harmful and can create ulceration of the mouth and face, not to mention hallucinations. Commercially-prepared powder and capsules are the best use of this strong herb.

A hard-to-grow tropical plant, not normally available for personal cultivation.

The rhizome, which is dried and peeled.

Kava kava is touted these days as an herb to use for nervousness and insomnia. It may help with muscle spasm and associated pain. Some people tout it as an alternative to traditional pain killers such as aspirin. Women may find it helpful for menopause symptoms. Kava kava also has mild diuretic effects and so may help with water retention, which then may also help in the treatment of rheumatism. Kava kava is being touted as a safe alternative to drugs such as Prozac and Valium. However, kava kava is also considered to have narcotic effects.

None noted and not recommended.

☞ Safest use is in capsule or powder form. Can be taken as a tea or drink.

Should be used only occasionally and only after advice from your physician or homeopath. Long term use has the potential to create liver problems. Should not be used with alcohol, by children, pregnant women, nursing mothers, individuals who suffer from depression or people taking medications for depression, anxiety, and other nervous disorders. Because of its sedative actions, driving after using kava kava should be avoided. A safer herb to use instead of kava kava may be chamomile.

Kelp

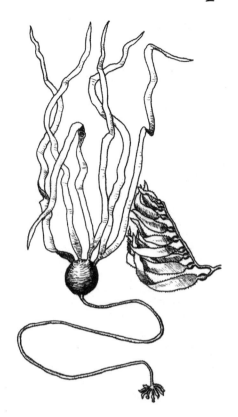

On trips to the Oregon coast, nothing is more pleasant than long walks on the beach together. My wife and I explore the beach, the rocks, find interesting pieces of driftwood to lug home. But we also notice long, cylindrical ocean plants, uprooted by the tides and permanently stranded on the beach. These "seaweeds" are often 12 feet long. We know them as kelp. Dark gray to green, it looks like a long tube an inch or so thick with a bulb and spinach-looking leaves on the end. Kelp is part of a family of sea plants often called "sea vegetables" or "ocean herbs" that have wonderful health benefits. Not covered here, but for you to consider, are *spirulina* and *chlorella*. Kelp is actually a giant-sized marine algae.

The whole plant, rich in iodine, B vitamins, other minerals and trace elements.

Considered brain food. Plus, kelp may help with the sensory nerves, the spinal cord, blood vessels, even finger- and toenails. Kelp may even help with a variety of conditions from hair loss to ulcers and is considered a safe digestive aid for constipation. Ocean herbs are considered detoxifiers for the body, helping rid the body of excess fluids and fatty wastes. There is also a belief that these sea vegetables are great protectors against environmental pollutants and radiation.

How about a seaweed bath to improve skin and hair tone and condition.

Ground, use as a salt substitute. In Asian cultures seaweed is consumed and prepared in the same way we may do green beans and carrots. You can consume much of these because they have no fat and low calories. These wonderful treats from the sea can also help in a weight loss program.

Can be eaten raw but is usually dried for medicinal purposes and then ground into powder. It is also found in liquid form as a health tonic.

Jonah found himself wrapped in seaweed just before the Lord provided a big fish to keep him from drowning and to teach him a lesson about obedience (Jon. 2:5). Maybe he should have taken a few bites of seaweed while it was available!

The sea is often symbolic of the troubles of humankind. The restless sea is a fine example of human lives without God, always in turmoil and problems.

Only one: If you have iodine-related thyroid problems, avoid kelp.

Lavender

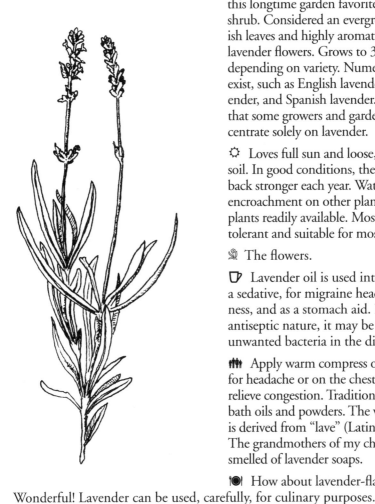

⊞ Originally from the Mediterranean, this longtime garden favorite is a perennial shrub. Considered an evergreen, it has grayish leaves and highly aromatic, purple or lavender flowers. Grows to 3 feet tall, depending on variety. Numerous varieties exist, such as English lavender, French lavender, and Spanish lavender. So popular, that some growers and garden societies concentrate solely on lavender.

☼ Loves full sun and loose, well-drained soil. In good conditions, the plant comes back stronger each year. Watch for encroachment on other plants. Seeds and plants readily available. Most are drought tolerant and suitable for most zones.

🌹 The flowers.

☕ Lavender oil is used internally as a sedative, for migraine headaches, dizziness, and as a stomach aid. Because of its antiseptic nature, it may be useful against unwanted bacteria in the digestive system.

⛲ Apply warm compress on the forehead for headache or on the chest to help relieve congestion. Traditionally used for bath oils and powders. The word "lavender" is derived from "lave" (Latin, "to wash"). The grandmothers of my childhood always smelled of lavender soaps.

🍽 How about lavender-flavored cookies? Wonderful! Lavender can be used, carefully, for culinary purposes.

☞ Cut the flowery stems at the height of the bloom and bunch them together. Let dry naturally. The pungent aroma will last for months and make a nice deodorizer for your home. To take internally, use drops of the oil or infuse the flowers or the leaves, picked before the flower blooms. Steep 1 teaspoon in ½ cup water.

📖 None noted. But one French herbalist described the scent of the lavender flower as "God's gift to earth." I agree. It's a heavenly scent sent from God. Perhaps we'll find lavender in Heaven. May each whiff of lavender remind us that our lives before God and before others should be a fragrance that will attract them to Christ's love. "Thanks be to God, who ... through us spreads everywhere the fragrance of the knowledge of him. For we are to God the aroma of Christ among those who are being saved and those who are perishing" (2 Cor. 2:15).

❗ This is a very strong herb, so use it carefully.

Licorice

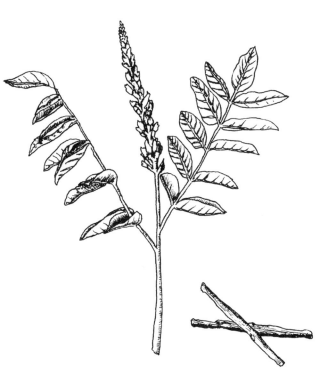

✺ Originating in Europe, varieties grow in North America. This herb is a perennial with woody stems, dark green foliage, and yellowish-to-purple flowers that bloom in the heart of summer. It grows from 3 to 6 feet tall.

☼ Propagate licorice from root sections. Grow it in rich, fine soil like what you might notice in a dry river bed. To grow it in pots, you will need ones that can provide up to 3 feet of depth for root development.

🌺 The root, harvested in the fall, in the fourth year of life.

☪ Licorice is a multi-use herb long favored in candies and sweets, but with many medicinal uses. Believed to have positive effects upon a woman's hormonal system and a strengthening and balancing effect upon the reproductive system. It may also have a regulating effect upon the kidneys and the adrenal glands. It may help people who are hypoglycemic or who suffer from diabetes. Licorice is used to relieve sore throats, coughs, laryngitis, bronchitis, and other similar complaints. Research is being done, because it is possible that licorice may even be a cancer fighter. If you are feeling stressed and exhausted, then try some licorice. But note alternatives (below) to the "licorice" candy that may actually be synthetic and certainly will contain refined white sugar or corn syrup.

🍴 Because the rootstock is sweet to the taste and it combines well with honey, consider using it as an alternative to sugar.

☞ You can make a syrup by simmering the roots for a few hours, then after discarding the root, combine the decoction with a little honey. To make a tea, steep 1 teaspoon rootstock in 1 cup water.

❗ If you have high blood pressure or heart problems, check with your physician before using licorice. Over use of licorice candy may cause some people to develop edema.

Lovage

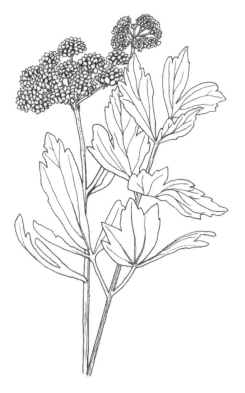

🏵 Love the lovage, just make sure it is the right one. The lovage described here is *Levisticum officinale*. This is a sweet and mild herb. A perennial, its leaves look a bit like oak leaves and the whole plant looks like giant celery. This is a Mediterranean plant that adapts well to cool climates, such as it has done in Great Britain where it can be found growing in the wild. Lovage can grow to 6 feet tall, has small white to pink and even yellow flowers that bloom in early summer. Note a strong but sweet aroma. This can be a fun addition to your herb garden, but it can be somewhat invasive.

☼ Grows easily enough from seed or by separating the rootstock. Likes sun, but is very adaptable. Needs adequate space.

🌹 Pretty much the whole plant, but most of the medicinal value comes from the root.

🍶 Lovage is a mild digestive aid. The ancient Romans and Greeks, and even Benedictine monks of the Middle Ages, ate the seeds as a digestive aid. Lovage was used for centuries as a tonic for the kidneys and bladder and even for ridding the body of kidney stones.

🛁 Leaves in the bath are a good skin conditioner. Essential oil is used for perfumes.

🍽 "Sharp and biting" is how the flavor is described. Often used as a substitute for pepper. The leaves add a sharp flavor to soups, stews, meats. Young shoots can be eaten raw like celery. The leaves can be used to make a tea with a pleasant and aromatic flavor. When baking bread or biscuits, try some lovage seeds sprinkled into the dough.

☞ The root can be dried and ground. Use leaves and seeds for culinary and medicinal purposes.

📖 None noted. But this plant has been used for millenniums, so it was probably known by the people of the biblical ages.

❗ Should not be used by pregnant women.

Mandrake

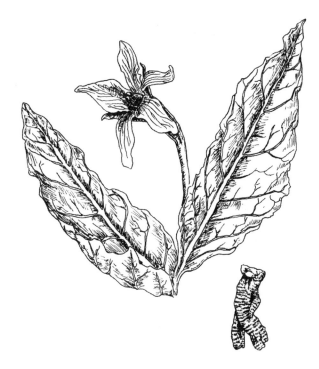

🏵 WARNING! This is a poisonous plant that should only be used as a prescription administered by a doctor. The mandrake plant that grows freely in North America is a different plant than the one that grows in the Bible lands. However, both plants are considered poisonous. I can give no recommendations for this plant.

🌺 The root.

🥤 🚹 🍽 Because of the danger of this plant, I will give no external, internal, or culinary suggestions. I list this herb because it is an herb of the Bible, but I mention it for no other reason than that.

📖 Genesis 30:14-16 tells of how Leah utilized the herb to help her conceive with Jacob. The mandrake root looks like lower human extremities and the superstition was that consuming the plant before sexual intercourse would help the woman to conceive. This odd story is a good example of willful people seeking superstition and other means to fulfill their desires rather than seeking God's help. Mandrakes are also called "love apples." But based upon the dangers of this plant, Leah was fortunate to have not died after consumption. The plant is also known as "devil's apples," which is a reminder of how Satan tempted Eve and Adam in the Garden of Eden and how their willful ways have shoved us all into a fallen world.

‼ Poisonous. Avoid using this plant.

Marjoram
(Oregano)

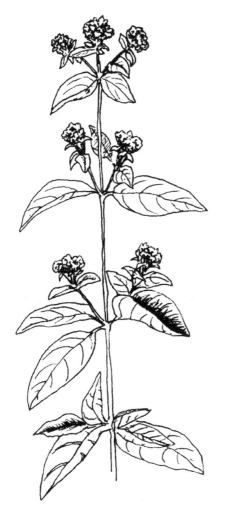

🏵 A favorite culinary herb specifically used in Italian- and Mediterranean-style cooking. While the flavors and appearance are nearly the same, the main difference between marjoram and oregano is that marjoram is more of a perennial. It has purple flowers from mid-summer to early fall. Oregano is an annual (climate depending). Both plants grow no taller than 12 inches.

☼ Easy to grow from seed, although slow to germinate. Loves sun. For those in the northern climates, this plant will be an annual, unless you can successfully grow it inside year round, which is not easy. I grow it year round with new plantings 2 to 4 times a year, and during the winter months keep it in my sunniest window.

🌿 The whole plant.

🍵 These herbs are beneficial for digestion, menstrual cycle and cramps, as well as repiratory ailments. The flowers are said to help with sea sickness and toothache.

👪 Breathe in the steam of a marjoram or oregano infusion to help clear your nose and respiratory passages when you have contracted a cold. You can also use it to treat a sore throat or mild mouth problems.

🍲 The greatest contribution of these herbs, in my mind, is what they do to spice up pasta, soups like minestrone, stews, any tomato dish, and Italian vegetables; and the sense of well-being they provide through aroma therapy while dinner is cooking and filling the house with wonderful smells.

☞ Fresh or dried, sprinkle into favorite recipes. To infuse as a tea, use 1 teaspoon herb per 1 cup water.

❗ May irritate the uterus during the menstrual cycle or in pregnant women. Check with your doctor.

Marsh Mallow

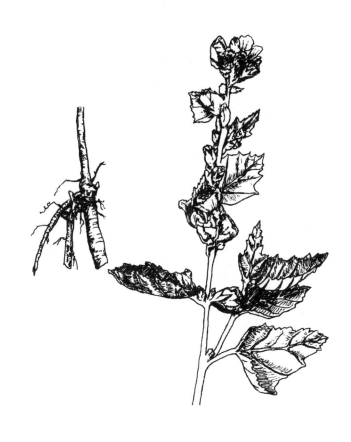

⊞ This is not the sweet confectionery that you roast over a campfire and squeeze between graham crackers and chocolate. Marsh mallow is a plant that will grow as a perennial or annual, depending upon the climate. Grows to 2 to 3 feet tall. Produces large, white and pinkish flowers.

☼ Easy enough to grow. Prefers a sandy or loose soil.

🌷 The whole plant.

🍵 If you are plagued with ulcers or colitis, then the marsh mallow plant may bring you some relief. Best method is to dry the leaves for a tea.

🏥 By making and applying a poultice of the herb, you may find that it helps to relieve the discomfort of skin irritations and inflammations.

🍽 Add new, tender leaves to salads.

☞ Soak 1 teaspoon marsh mallow leaves in ½ cup water; let stand for up to 8 hours, then heat to bath temperature. Don't boil.

📖 This plant is found in and around the Dead Sea and is also known there as "salt plant" because of its salty taste. There are many varieties and sub-species of the plant, so the one you may buy at your garden shop is probably different than what you may find in the Bible lands. Job 30:4 reads, "In the brush they gathered salt herbs." In this passage, marsh mallow is described as a food with little palatability.

Meadowsweet

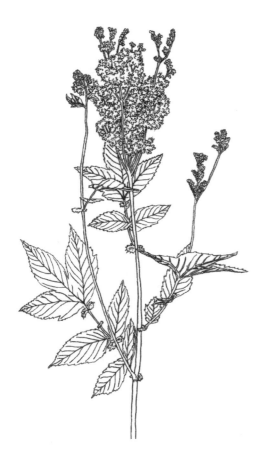

⌘ What a lovely name for a plant and apropos to all of its benefits. Meadowsweet is a common wildflower native to Europe, now being cultivated because of its mild qualities. This is a plant that can be found in moist areas in the U.S., growing wild from the east to the midwest, evidently brought over by colonists. Look for fern-like, graceful dark-green foliage and delicate cream-colored flowers. The plant grows from 2 to 4 feet tall. Meadowsweet smells just as you would hope it would—sweet and pleasant.

✿ Needs a moist to boggy, non-acid soil, sun to partial sun. Seeds are readily available. Establish it in your garden and it will self-sow.

🌺 Rootstock, flowers, leaves.

🍵 While this herb has been used for millenniums, in this new millennium meadowsweet is becoming quite popular because of its array of medicinal benefits and its mildness and safety.

It is very beneficial for the digestive system from indigestion, gas, ulcers, hiatal hernia, upset bowels and diarrhea. It has a cleansing tonic effect upon the whole digestive system, top to bottom. Meadowsweet is one of the natural substances in which we would find salicylates or those substances used to make aspirin, so it has recently been touted as a natural form of pain relief. The herb has anti-inflammatory properties that help with arthritis, gout, swollen joints, headaches, neuralgia, back pain and other aches and pains. Meadowsweet is also mildly diuretic so it may help with high blood pressure and even provide relief from skin rashes.

👫 A decoction can be helpful as an eyewash.

🍽 Use the flowers for beverages. Include them the next time you make sun tea. The leaves are used to flavor soups and stews.

☞ One ounce of the dried herb infused in a pint of water. With a little bit of honey, meadowsweet has a very pleasant flavor. Collect the herb when it flowers.

❣ No concerns noted. This seems to be a very safe herb similar to chamomile.

Mint

(Spearmint   Peppermint   Apple Mint   ... etc.)

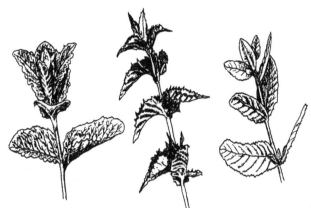

⊞ Probably no other herb is used more than this one, from your favorite chewing gum and candies, to the toothpaste and mouthwash you use in the morning. The plant is a perennial that dies out during winter, but reseeds itself naturally. The plant grows 2 to 3 feet tall. Purple and blue flowers appear July to September.

✿ Prospers in most soils, although dry, loose soils are best. Will grow abundantly and will quickly take over, so plant in a contained space or in large bottomless pots.

🌺 The leaves.

🗓 Consider mint next time you need an antacid. Peppermint tea or candy work well for mild heartburn and indigestion. I have not used antacids for many years, but was addicted to them at one time. These strong medicines can be harsh remedies, and I fear can do more long-term damage than good. Some antacids can actually promote more problems. Mint helps to stabilize your stomach. Try combinations or rotations of mint and chamomile and you may discover, after a time, you have fewer problems with indigestion. Also, try mint as a healthy alternative to coffee.

Herb specialist Earl Mindell suggests using mint as an alternative to aspirin or acetaminophen. He says to drink a strong cup of mint tea, then lie down for a short time, and you may find your headache goes away without having to resort to the medicine cabinet.

⫶ The leaves have a cooling effect on skin irritations.

🍽 Other than the obvious for teas and drinks, try tender leaves chopped into salads or sprinkled on yogurt or ice cream. They add a great flavor.

☞ Pour 1 cup boiling water over 2-3 teaspoons fresh or dried mint leaves, and steep. Peppermint oil is also available in local stores that carry herbs.

📖 Considered a bitter herb, mint would be used during Passover celebrations. It is mentioned as an offering to God in Matthew 23:23.

❗ No cautionary concerns noted, but mint is a strong herb.

Mugwort

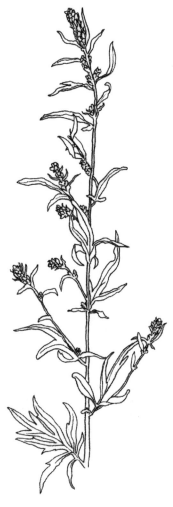

⊞ Mugwort is a common plant or weed found throughout the Americas, Europe, and Asia. Specifically in America it grows more in the east but the plant is available in all parts of the country, so don't be surprised to find one growing in the wild as an escapee from someone's garden. A tall plant, it will grow from 1 to 5 feet tall. Notice smooth gray green to dark green leaves with a downy appearance on the under leaf. Appearance is similar to wormwood. Small, non-descript flowers in reddish, greenish to pale yellow colors.

☼ Grows like a weed and is adaptable to most soils. Can be grown from seed or by dividing an existing plant. Mugwort makes for an interesting contrast in the garden, but it can be invasive.

🌱 Specifically the rootstock, but the whole herb is also used.

▽ Mugwort is considered an appetite stimulator and a nerve calmative, and it has diuretic properties. It is said to help with menstruation regulation. Chinese herbalists prescribe mugwort for rheumatism symptoms.

👥 An old Roman legend indicates that putting the leaves in one's shoes prevents aching feet. Roman soldiers would do this on long marches. Juice from the plant can be used as a treatment for poison oak and as an insect repellent. In fact, mugwort's name comes from an old English word, "moughte," meaning moth.

In olden days it was used to keep moths away from stored woolen garments.

🍽 Some find the slightly bitter flavor a good addition to stuffing, used as you might use sage. It has been used as a tea substitute.

☞ Dried rootstock for tea, the leaves for culinary purposes or in your shoes.

📖 Mugwort has a connection with John the Baptist in that it was thought by the medievals that he wore a girdle of mugwort to help sustain him in the desert. Mugwort was also used to ward off evil spirits, the devil himself, and traveling salesmen. I will let you decide which you would think the worse.

❗ Excessive doses can be considered poisonous. Plants in this family have a toxic nature and should be used and handled carefully.

Mullein
(Common)

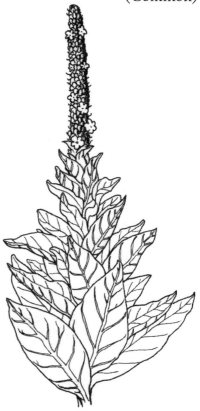

🏵 *Verbascum thapsus.* For years I have noticed this plant. Mullein seems to grow everywhere in the West regardless of the climate. But it's everywhere else in the country as well. I used to think it was some odd wild corn the way the stocks grew. Common mullein can grow to heights of 8 feet on a thick stem that sprouts a foot-long flower that looks like a cornhusk with the corn exposed. The plant has large light-green leaves and the plant loves to sprout along dirt paths and old roads.

☼ This weed will probably sprout up in your yard if you let it. Very drought tolerant. A number of varieties exist. For your garden you may consider purple-flowered *dumulosum,* a dwarf variety or *phoeniceum.* It takes 2 years to fully develop.

🌹 Leaves and flowers.

☞ Long used for colds and respiratory complaints, it is said to provide relief for digestive ailments. The flower, infused as a tea, is said to help with pain and to aid sleep. Oil derived from the flower is said to help relieve earaches.

👥 The flowers, used in a vapor, may relieve congestion and a stuffy nose. The leaves are said to help in the removal of warts and may help heal wounds and sores. The flowers have been used as a hair dye for those who want to be blonde. And I've heard that young Amish women, who are not allowed to use make-up, will take the leaves and rub them on their cheeks to get a blush effect.

☞ A decoction made from the root, leaves, and flowers.

📖 From Bible times, it is said that Agrippa indicated that the fragrance of the plant had an overpowering effect upon demons. Whether this is attributed to the first or the second Herod Agrippa, I don't know. Of course, the first was the evil adulterer who had John the Baptist beheaded. The second was the king, or ruler, that Paul stood before to argue his case. He said, after Paul's long discourse, "Do you think that in such a short time, you can persuade me to become a Christian?" (Acts 26:28). Whether this Agrippa ever became a Christian we will not know on this side of Heaven. If he did, he didn't need mullein to deal with the demons. When we accept Jesus as Savior, then the demons quake in their boots.

❗ The seeds are considered toxic and should not be used.

Mustard

(Black, White, and other varieties)

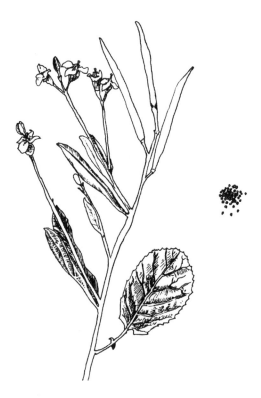

⚘ An annual plant found worldwide in many varieties. Can grow to 7 feet tall. Yellow flowers grow first and then are replaced by pods containing many seeds.

☼ Grows easily. Fooled by the small size of the seeds, I always grow too much mustard.

🌾 Leaves and seeds.

🗢 Mustard greens help keep the digestive system operating smoothly, aid proper bowel function. High in fiber. The seeds have been used to treat chronic constipation.

👪 Mustard plasters were common medical practice a century ago to help clear the bronchi in flu or bronchitis sufferers.

🍲 Young, tender mustard leaves are great in salads. More mature ones can be cooked like spinach. Eat the stems fresh from the garden, and a hot flavor will zing your palette and clear your nasal passages. Dry and grind the seeds, then mix them with vinegar to make your own spreadable mustard.

☞ For plasters use ground, black mustard seeds and water to make a thick paste, wrap in linen and apply to area to be treated.

📖 The Bible teaches about the mustard seed and how it grows to be the biggest plant in the garden. You can see this is true when you compare the size of the seed with the size of the plant that grows from it. There are many varieties of mustard. Some are like trees, and that is why Jesus said that even the birds could rest in them.

Mark 4:32 uses the mustard seed in a parable about the faith that we can develop. God gives us faith as a little seed to be watered and nourished by the Holy Spirit. The plant grows profusely and is a great reminder of how a little seed of faith can grow in us to give us a great faith in knowing that "faith is being sure of what we hope for and certain of what we do not see" (Heb. 11:1). See more about mustard in the "Jesus and the Herbs" section of this book.

❗ This is a very strong herb. Heavy use can inflame the digestive system. A compress put directly on the skin can cause a rash or redness. (This may be soothed with olive oil.) People who are anemic or who have ulcers should avoid mustard.

Myrrh

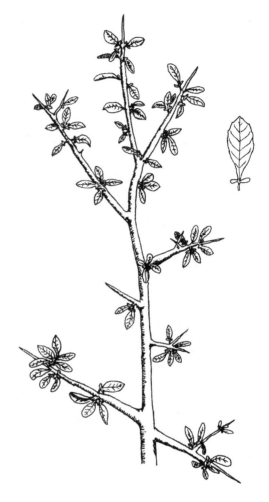

▣ Sap drawn from the gum myrrh tree. Similar to frankincense and one of the trio of gifts given by the Magi to the baby Jesus, myrrh has high spiritual significance.

☼ None noted. But you may be able to purchase seeds or plants from herb growers that specialize in exotics.

✑ The sap.

℧ Myrrh has been used as a stomach tonic and to treat halitosis. It can be used as a mouth wash or gargle for sore throat, painful teeth and gums, possibly even asthma. Studies have indicated myrrh may help build the immune system like the highly-touted echinacea.

⁜ It is used as an antiseptic, astringent, or as a douche.

☞ Used for cosmetic purposes and as a perfume. Purchase myrrh powder.

In the days before embalming, myrrh was used in the preparation of the deceased body.

📖 The uniqueness of myrrh as a gift for a newborn babe is interesting. You know the story. The wisemen came bearing gifts of gold, frankincense, and myrrh. We can understand that gold represents Jesus as King, and frankincense represents Jesus as God, but what about the myrrh? In those days, myrrh was an expensive substance usually bought for the purpose of burial. So why give a child, at the beginning of his life, something that would be used at the end of his life? Myrrh represented Jesus as the sacred sacrifice, the Lamb of God who would die to take away our sins. If you ever have an opportunity to use myrrh, may it remind you, in solemn celebration, that he died for you. In healing services, I sometimes use myrrh oil as a reminder to those who seek healing that "by his wounds we are healed" (Isa. 53:5).

❗ High doses are considered poisonous. People who have kidney problems, and pregnant women need to check with their physician before using myrrh.

Nasturtium

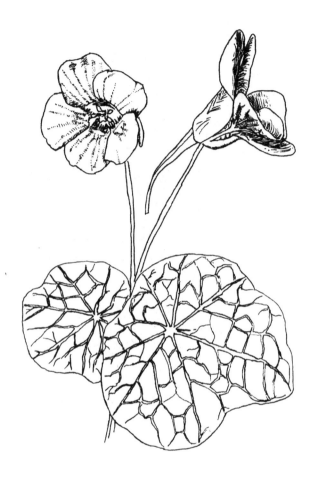

⊞ Another beauty for the flower bed with its prolific red, orange, and yellow flowers. Native to South America. Grows as an annual.

☼ In colder climates this flower really only prospers in the summer and is very sensitive to frost. Sow directly into the ground because it is very hard to transplant.

✿ Flowers, leaves, and seeds.

⛉ Nasturtium is good as an antiseptic and for breaking up congestion in the respiratory system. Nasturtium is reportedly beneficial as a blood builder.

ﺉﻔﻔ Nasturtium has antiseptic qualities, so the juice can be used as a disinfectant.

🍽 Garnish your next salad with fresh-cut nasturtium petals. Also try making nasturtium jelly.

☞ For culinary use, sprinkle the flowers on salads, etc. For internal use, the juice of the nasturtium is available at herb shops.

Nettle
(Stinging)

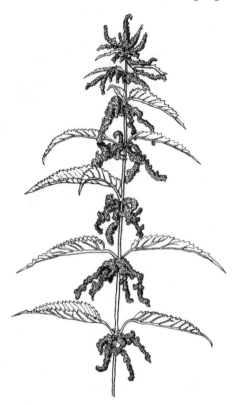

One day while fishing in a lake I thought I spotted wild mint growing by the shore. I pulled off a leaf and put it to my nose expecting to get a whiff of refreshing mint. That's not what I got. I thought maybe a bee had been hiding under the leaf, because my fingers and lips felt like they had been stung. I thus had the displeasure of meeting stinging nettle. So I was surprised one day to find nettle being sold in my local nutrition store. The plant grows as a wild perennial, reaching 7 feet tall. It has serrated pointy leaves, downy underneath. But don't let the appearance fool you, because these downy hairs do the stinging. It blooms small greenish flowers mid-summer to early fall.

☼ Carefully! Wear gloves. I think I'll use a derived product from the store.

🌹 The plant.

� This herb has great benefits. The juice can be used for digestive problems, urinary concerns, and to stimulate the production of milk in nursing mothers. It is also said to help with a number of disorders experienced by women. Be cautious with this herb, though. In fact, the best way to use it is in a form processed by a professional who knows how to handle the stinging plant.

☞ Get the safe and processed material at the store.

📖 The Bible mentions nettles and thorny plants. Isaiah 34:13 mentions Edom becoming overrun by nettles and brambles, a place that no one but jackals would want to go. My first encounter reminded me of the story of the fall of mankind in Genesis. There was an idyllic paradise, and then because of man's disobedience God placed a curse on his creation that still exists today. God cursed the ground, plants changed and some became dangerous. "It will produce thorns and thistles for you" (Gen. 3:18). In Eden, I can imagine, a rose bush had no thorns. Now the nettle has qualities that are beneficial and yet attributes that can harm. Nettles, thorns and such always remind me that while there may be great beauty in this world, there remains a curse on it and we have no one to blame but ourselves. But for those who love and seek God, who have sought the Savior for forgiveness and the path of life, eventually we will live in a world where no curse will make life painful again.

❗ Old plants are considered poisonous.

Nutmeg
(also Mace)

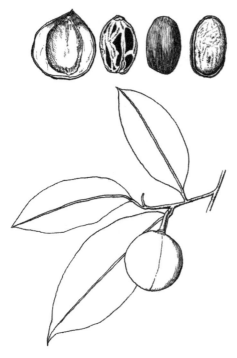

⌗ I have included a number of traditional culinary spices. These also are herbs and well known to most people because of their culinary value, but you may not know of their medicinal values. Nutmeg comes from an evergreen tree (*Myristica fragrans*) found in the tropics of the West Indies, in parts of South Africa, the Molucca Islands, and is now cultivated in India and Brazil. The nutmeg tree can grow to heights of 25 to 40 feet. It has a grayish-brown smooth bark, leaves 1 inch long that are a glossy dark green. The flowers are small, inconspicuous and yellow in color. The ground spice you buy is from the nut of this tree. It actually provides two spices: from the membrane of the nut comes mace and from the kernel of the nut, nutmeg. In the west, nutmeg is not to be confused with an evergreen tree known as California nutmeg that produces a similar-looking nut.

☼ Nutmeg trees need tropical, high humidity with rich soil, shady-to-part-shady conditions, and temperatures that never dip below 64 degrees. For us in the states, that means that we have to grow one in a greenhouse.

🌿 The kernel, dried and ground into powder. Essential oils are also used.

♉ Nutmeg has a calming effect upon the stomach and it may stimulate the appetite. Simply smelling the pleasant aroma can make one's mouth water. It is believed to improve digestion and relieve the discomfort of nausea and excess gas. Nutmeg is also said to help with insomnia.

👪 Like oil of clove, nutmeg oil can help with a toothache. It can also be rubbed onto the skin for aches and pains. Moderation is important.

🍽 Pretty much endless when it comes to baking and cooking.

☞ Grind into powder or press oil.

📖 Wherever spices are mentioned in the Bible, nutmeg certainly could have been one of them.

❗ John Lust, author of *The Herb Book,* and other authorities indicate that nutmeg has hallucinogenic properties similar to mescaline, and eating of the whole nut is poisonous and can actually lead to death.

Oak
(White)

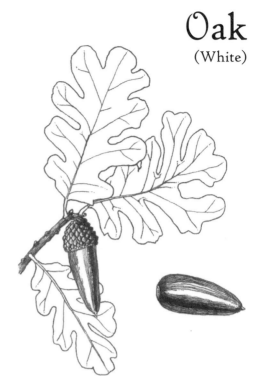

⌕ This tree grows in most places in the U.S. While there are many varieties of oak, it is the bark of the white oak that has the herbal benefits that we include here. Oaks, of course, are easily identified by their familiar leaves, gnarly bark, and acorns.

☼ Pretty much grows anywhere. Oak grows slowly and will take up a lot of room when mature, reaching heights of 60 to 150 feet.

⚘ The bark and the acorn.

𝌆 An infusion or tea of the bark is said to help many conditions: menstrual problems, kidney and bladder infections. There are reports that oak bark can help with varicose veins, reduction of fever, and even stemming internal hemorrhages.

⍫ Externally, oak has antiseptic and astringent qualities and can be used as a wash for skin irritations, sores, sore throat, as a douche, and to treat hemorrhoids. A foot bath of oak bark is said to be very rejuvenating for tired, sore feet.

⦿ I raised pigs once and they loved acorns. They obviously do not have the discriminating palate that humans have. Acorns are considered edible if you can handle the bitter taste. However, if you really want to try them, then you will want to boil them (kernels only) until the water is clear. Some old-timers will take the nut and roll it in a sugar syrup, thus making a kind of acorn candy. The nut can also be ground into flour, which can be used for breads and is evidently quite excellent.

☞ Steep the bark in boiling water for up to 30 minutes.

📖 A number of Bible verses refer to the oak of the Bible lands. We often think of it as the "mighty oak," a tree that is strong and sturdy and withstands much to grow large, wide, and old. However, the oak, as with anything else, including each of us, is no match for the power of God. "The voice of the Lord is powerful; the voice of the Lord is majestic" (Ps. 29:4). This powerful voice breaks cedars, flashes forth lightning, and shakes deserts. Even the mighty oak is no match. "The voice of the Lord twists the oaks and strips the forests bare" (Ps. 29:9). Isn't it amazing to think that the cares and noise of this world can get so much in our way, that we miss the powerful, and yet still, small voice of the Lord. We, however, who know God, through his son, glory in his voice. And in his temple we will cry, "Holy is the Lord." While his mighty voice could destroy the world, he will bless his people with peace. The mighty oak can be a reminder to us of the mighty voice of God, the same God who brings us peace. Are you listening today?

Oat

and Oat Straw

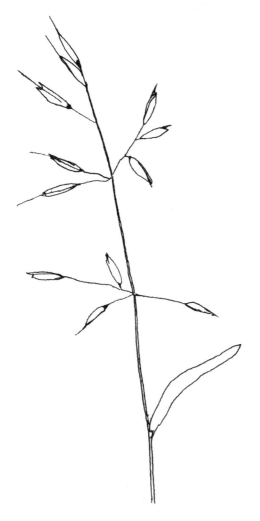

🏵 An annual grass grown for the grain. Oat grows 2 to 4 feet. Pale green leaves and clusters of flowers develop into grain at the end of the season.

☼ None noted. But you may want to try growing some in a small section as an ornamental, and then harvest it.

🌱 Grain and straw.

🍵 Oat acts as a stimulant and enhances the mood. Have you ever noticed after eating a bowl of oatmeal or an oatmeal cookie that you feel a sense of satisfaction? Oat could be part of the reason. Folks suffering from stomach ills and dyspepsia will find oat soothing. Oat straw, infused in a tea, is said to help with congestion problems. And of course, oats and oat bran are said to help lower cholesterol. Oat is a tonic for the nerves and a good source of vitamin B.

👫 Oat seems to have many external benefits as well. The straw can be used in baths to help soothe the skin, soothe hemorrhoids and rheumatic conditions, and relieve aching feet after a hard day. Use topically to treat flaky skin, frostbite, chilblains, and wounds. Cosmetically, oat is used to make women more beautiful by improving and revitalizing the skin.

🍽 Many. For breakfast consider passing on the tiger, the captain, the pebbles, the puffs, and the pops; and get back to breakfast the way it ought to be—oatmeal. In baking, consider substituting oat flour for processed white flour.

📖 Boil small pieces of oat grain or straw for an hour. Or just add oatmeal into a bath. Oat oil is also available at health food stores.

Olive

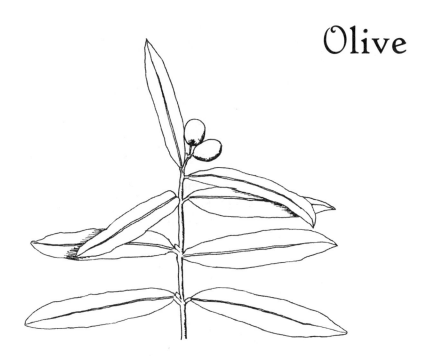

⚜ While I am very familiar with the olive fruit—Thanksgiving dinner wouldn't be the same without them, and Italian dishes wouldn't be the same without the oil that is pressed from the fruit—I was not aware that the leaves and the bark from the tree also have great benefit. And certainly, as we consider the olive, we will also find much spiritual benefit. The olive tree is considered an evergreen whose origins are the lands of the Bible—the Mediterranean and the tropics. Visit California, Southern Arizona, and other warmer parts of the U.S., and you will find olive orchards in abundance. The trees, reaching up to 25 feet, are distinctive in appearance with the gnarled bark, dark-green and silvery leaves, fragrant white flowers, and oblong fruit.

☼ To grow olives, you need to live in a dryer, warmer climate, where temperatures never get below 15°F. If you live in a northern area, try growing an olive tree in a pot that you can bring inside during winter. Many varieties are available, including fruitless ones for landscaping and a smaller variety called "skylark dwarf."

🌱 Leaves, bark, and fruit.

℧ First and foremost, olive oil is one of the few vegetable oils that is actually beneficial for you. Because it's high in monounsaturated fat, it has high potential for lowering dangerous cholesterol levels, while not reducing beneficial cholesterol. A steady diet of this marvelous oil reduces the incidence of heart disease. Olive oil's properties aid in digestion and normal bowel function. Drinking a tea made of a decoction or infusion of olive leaves and inner bark is said to be good for treating fever and nervousness.

(Olive continued on next page)

♔ For treating dry hair and scalp. As antiseptic and conditioner for the skin. For use on burns, bruises, insect bites, sprains, and itchy skin.

🍽 Use in any dish that calls for oil, as a great alternative. (I'm a popcorn addict, and I've gone to cooking popcorn in a little olive oil. It doesn't take much; adds great taste to the corn; and I like knowing that it is good for me.)

☞ Use the oil liberally. Use bark and leaves at a ratio of 1 or 2 teaspoons per 1 cup water.

📖 The olive fruit and trees are mentioned nearly 60 times in the Bible. The symbol (for peace) of a dove carrying an olive branch comes from the story of Noah and the worldwide flood that destroyed the antediluvian world. "When the dove returned to him [Noah] in the evening, there in its beak was a freshly plucked olive leaf! Then Noah knew that the water had receded from the earth" (Gen. 8:11). Only Noah and his family were found fit to be saved. God commanded Noah to build a huge ark and all the birds and land animals were placed on the ark. The earth was destroyed because of the wickedness of the people. But when the water receded, God set a rainbow in the clouds and made a peace pact with humankind.

Peace should have ruled—once you have peace with God, then peace is obtainable with others. But soon man disobeyed God and became violent again. Now a different end awaits the earth—destruction by fire. Man chooses to break the peace with God; and God will not put up with it forever. But the peace pact is still available to all who will seek it. Christ is our peace, which we receive when we accept him as Lord and Savior. He gives a new kind of inner peace—not an enforced peace—in the knowing that all is at rest between the Savior and those who need to be saved.

In Jesus' parable of the ten virgins (see Matt. 25:1-13), ten maidens went in search of the bridegroom, but five of the virgins brought no olive oil to replenish their lamps, so they missed his arrival. The oil is a reminder to us that we must be watchful and waiting for Jesus' second coming.

Olive oil is symbolic of the healing ministry of the Holy Spirit. In healing services, olive oil is preferred for anointing the sick. In prayer, asking of the Holy Spirit, we seek healing for those who are ill or injured.

Christians—gentile believers in Jesus—are described by Paul in Romans 11:17 as a wild olive shoot, grafted in among the others, sharing in the nourishing sap of the olive tree; a humble reminder that we become the children of God not by anything we can do, but by grace alone. In the Garden of Gethsemene (which means "olive press") Jesus prayed and sweat blood, but said to Father God, "Thy will, not my will be done." He accepted the cross, so that we could be grafted into his love forever.

❢ The only thing I noted in my research was that pregnant women should avoid using olive oil as a laxative.

Onion
(and Leeks)

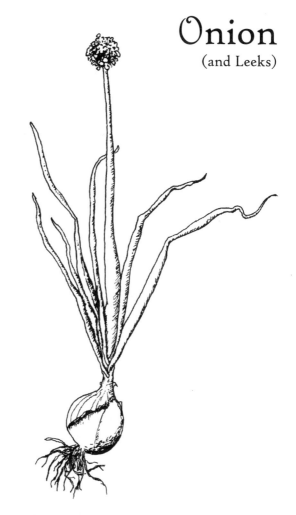

▦ A most common staple, the onion offers quite a bit to the healing herb garden.

☼ Plant by seeds or sets (small onion plants) year round in most climates. Prefers a dryer, loose soil for proper bulb development. Too much water will cause the onion to rot. Onion is one of the few plants in your vegetable garden that prefers less, not more, water.

⚘ The bulb.

♉ Onion has health benefits similar to those of garlic and chives. It certainly aids in proper digestion. It also helps to eliminate problems such as bacteria in the gastrointestinal tract. There seem to be benefits for the heart and the regulation of blood pressure. Onion is also said to help sexual potency. And this may surprise you, but it may help to curb heartburn. Onion juice mixed with honey is good for coughs, a scratchy throat, and as an expectorant.

ⵜ Apply to the skin as a daily cure for athlete's foot, warts, and liver spots. Like garlic, onion may help in the fight against stomach cancer. This most readily available herb is beneficial in many ways.

🍽 I don't eat much red meat because it seems to slow down my digestive system. But on the rare occasions I do have a steak, I smother it in onions. Not only do the onions make the steak taste better, they also help it pass through my digestive system more quickly.

📖 This is another vegetable that the nation of Israel complained about not having when God sent them on a journey through the wilderness, on their way to the Promised Land. Have you heard the expression, "The more you complain, the longer God lets you live"? In the case of the complaining Hebrews, the more they complained, the longer they got to wander in the desert. It's nice to know that if we truly trust God, we will see more blessings.

❗ If you are a nursing mother, eating onions may cause your baby to have colic.

Parsley

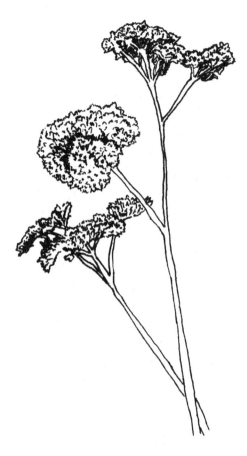

⚘ A biennial plant usually grown as an annual. It grows to a height of 6 to 12 inches and has bright, curly green leaves. The plant develops small white flowers, and then seeds.

☼ Grows easily enough from seed, although slow to germinate. It is one of those nice herbs that grows well in the garden mixed in with basil, tomatoes, and other Italian vegetables. Parsley is a very attractive plant, so try growing it in and around flowers, and you may notice the bugs stay away. Or grow it in an inside window box year-round.

🌹 Plant and seeds.

🍵 When you order at the restaurant, and they garnish your plate with a sprig of parsley, eat it. Full of vitamins A and C, plus calcium, thiamin, riboflavin, and niacin, it is good for you. If you are somewhat anemic, then there is added benefit. Because parsley is full of chlorophyll, it is a natural breath deodorizer. Parsley is a good digestive aid. It has a diuretic effect, so may help with the liver, kidney stones, and in normalizing blood pressure. Parsley tea or juice may be beneficial in treating dropsy, jaundice, asthma, and coughs.

👪 Parsley can be used as a poultice for nursing mothers suffering from swollen breasts. Also, utilize an infusion as a skin lotion or shampoo.

🍽 It cooks with anything and is good fresh, diced into a salad, or added to tuna or chicken salad. The culinary uses are considerable.

📖 Not specifically mentioned in the Bible, but since it is considered a "bitter herb," parsley may have been—and is today—used in Passover meals.

❗ It is suggested that pregnant women and people with kidney problems avoid parsley.

Passionflower

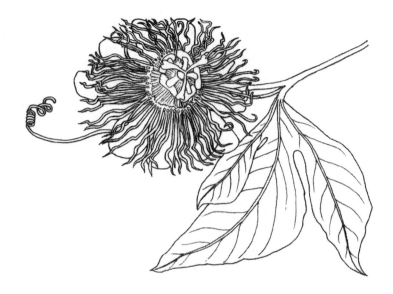

🏵 Specifically, *Passiflora incarnata*. Take a long look at the flower and you will get a good idea of how the name came about. This is an exciting herb to include in this book not only because of what it can do for you but also for its great spiritual significance. The passionflower is indigenous to the tropic and sub-tropic areas of the Americas, specifically here in the U.S. from Virginia, south and east to Texas. The root is perennial, meaning that the plant will come back each year. It is a large plant that can grow to 25 feet. This is a climbing plant with uniquely colored leaves of green and white and the beautiful cream-colored and/or lavender flowers. The flowers offer a sweet scent. The plant also produces an orange-colored berry that, when ripe, is as large as a chicken egg. The pulp in the berry is edible.

✿ There are numerous varieties of this plant and you may find just the right one for your growing zone. This is a vigorously growing plant, and for a plant found in tropical and semi-tropical areas, it's quite hardy. The passionflower is good to grow as a hedge, ground cover, and for arbors and other places you would like a vine-like plant to cascade and hang.

🌾 The whole plant.

⚱ This plant's claim to fame is its safe and effective tranquilizing properties. If you suffer from insomnia, anxiety, muscle tension and spasm, frayed nerves, plus headaches caused by stress and tension, then passionflower may be for you and a perhaps safer medicinal than over-the-counter or prescribed medicines designed by man to do the same.

🍽 The fruit can be eaten fresh or its juice used for a beverage.

(Passionflower continued on next page)

☞ Best to use capsules, teas, or tinctures professionally prepared.

📖 The name, passionflower, does not come from legends regarding romantic love and ardor but rather the trial, scourging, crown-of-thorns and crucifixion of he who paid the price for our sins, Jesus the Christ. His passion for us, his desire to not lose us to sin, is what is represented in this beautiful and intricate flower. The fascinating thing is that this plant wouldn't have been known to those who lived in the Bible lands. Yet its spiritual significance is most profound. The passionflower is named because parts of the blossom actually look like the crown of thorns, as well as the people, other implements and objects that make up the crucifixion story. And the final moments of the Passion of Our Lord and Savior, Jesus Christ are here, in this flower.

Spanish Catholic priests/missionaries to South America used the passionflower for teaching "The Calvary Lesson." Note that the flower petals look like the ring of thorns that were placed upon Christ's head. The ovary suggests a picture of the hammer. The three styles, often darkest in color, look like the three spikes that would have held Jesus to the cross—two through his wrists and one large one through his ankles or feet. The five anthers or stamens are symbolic of the five specific wounds that Christ received—three from the spikes, one from the crown and scourging, and the last one from the spear that pierced his side. There are ten sepals, those points farthest out on the flower, that are said to represent 10 disciples (not 12, because two, Judas and Peter, betrayed the Lord). Peter, of course, sought forgiveness, was reinstated, and is considered the earthly father of the Christian church.

What remains fascinating to me is how this plant was initially found only in the Americas, a place that was not evangelized for Christ for nearly sixteen centuries after his death and resurrection. Upon finding this flower, the priests realized they had an extraordinary evangelistic tool. The natives loved the nut of the flower and so the priests would take the opportunity to explain the ministry of Christ to them through the flower. God gives us examples in creation. (For instance, I often use the egg to explain the Trinity or triune nature of God.) Jesus taught using parables and the passionflower is one of the best living parables that teaches about Christ's dying and undying love for humankind.

I say, "Thank-you, Lord, for creating such a striking flower and such a fascinating way to remember and teach what you did for us."

"As for man, his days are like grass, he flourishes like a flower of the field; the wind blows over it and it is gone, and its place remembers it no more. But from everlasting to everlasting the Lord's love is with those who fear him" (Ps. 103:15-17a).

❣ If you are pregnant, check with your doctor before using passionflower. Also, a person should not drive or operate machinery while using passionflower.

Pennyroyal

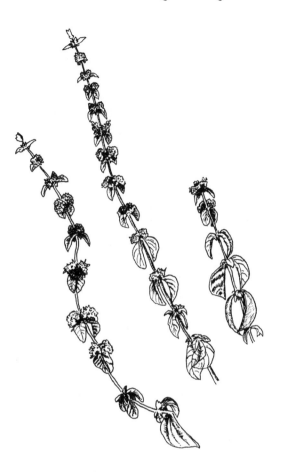

✿ A member of the mint family, pennyroyal is a pretty plant with a lovely and unique flower. An annual with lovely round leaves that grow up to 18 inches. Small clusters of lavender and purple flowers bloom from early summer to early fall. The whole plant has a sweet aromatic to pungent odor that some people find disagreeable.

✿ English or European pennyroyal makes a nice addition next to your water garden. The North American relative prefers a dryer area, but this is more of a shade-loving plant. In the wild, though, it seems to be tolerant of about anything and can be invasive and a bane to hay farmers and cattle ranchers.

✿ The whole plant.

✿ Pennyroyal has benefits similar to mint and is a digestive aid. It is said to be good for headaches and menstrual concerns.

✿ The leaves can be used as an external wash for skin problems, rashes, and itching. Pennyroyal is also commercially prepared and sold as an insect repellent. This may be its best use.

✿ A small dash on a salad may be suitable; but this is a very strong herb.

☞ To prepare as a tea, use 1 teaspoon of the herb per 1 cup boiling water.

❣ The oil of the pennyroyal should never be used internally. It should never be used externally except as an insect repellent. It should not be taken when pregnant, because it can cause miscarriage. Women who have tried to self abort with pennyroyal have died. Planned or unplanned, a child is a gift from God and deserves to have a life. Frankly, this plant makes me nervous. I like to grow the plants because they are so pretty, but I would only use pennyroyal in a processed form from an accredited herbalist.

Pomegranate

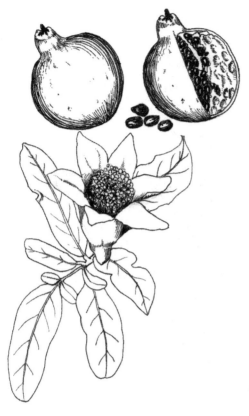

❊ Being a northerner, I once visited the farm country near San Diego and was fooled by a lovely tree full of what looked like large red apples. However, upon closer inspection, I discovered they were not apples but pomegranates. I'm not the only one who has been fooled, since another name for this wonderful fruit is "seeded apple." I include pomegranate because of its herbal qualities and spiritual significance. Pomegranate grows to 15-20 feet high. Dark brown bark. Green leaves. Large crimson-red flowers.

✿ Semi-tropical. Native of Asia but now found in the Mediterranean and the semi-tropical West of the U.S. In other areas, dwarf varieties have been grown to be kept inside during the winter months. For full development of the fruit you need much sun and an alkaline soil, and once established the tree is very drought tolerant.

🌿 The whole plant, for numerous uses.

🝑 For millenniums the rind and the leaves, with their astringent properties, have been used to treat patients with tapeworms. Eating the fruit may help with diarrhea.

👪 The rind can be helpful to the skin and for irritations of the throat and mouth. The flower is used as a dye, and the bark for the tanning of leather.

🍽 Enjoy this unique, sweet fruit. The juice is good as a drink mixed with other cooling beverages or for making wonderful, beautiful jelly and sauces.

☞ As a fruit, fresh. For the medicinal purposes of ridding of a tapeworm the leaves and rind are dried. Check with an acknowledged herbalist before using.

📖 Pomegranate symbolizes abundance and fruitfulness because hundreds of seeds are found in the fruit, enough to plant a huge orchard. The lovers in Song of Solomon enjoyed the fruit and nectar both physically and figuratively, I suppose. However, most intriguing is the use of the design of the pomegranate in the Jews' priestly clothing. At the hem of the blue knee-length robe, gold-, red-, and blue-colored pomegranates hung alternately with golden bells. The sweet taste of the fruit symbolizes the pleasantness of God's promises.

Pygeum

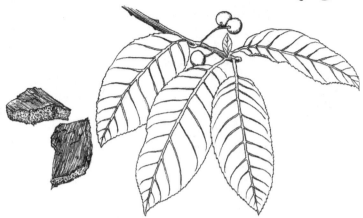

⚘ Pygeum is considered one of the new "miracle" herbs for men with benign prostate enlargement or BPH (benign prostatic hyperplasia). Pygeum has the promising potential of shrinking the enlarged prostate. The medicinal herb comes predominately from the bark of the African prune tree, *pygeum africanum* or its newer name, *prunus africana*. This evergreen tree grows in the higher elevations of Central and Southern Africa. A large, slow growing tree with dark brownish to gray bark, thick oblong leaves, cream-colored flowers, and fruit that resembles cherry. The tree is hardwood and used in furniture making. Pygeum has become a very popular product very quickly and there are numerous reports that this explosion of interest is causing an ecological nightmare with the harvesting of these trees. Some experts are so worried that they fear extinction could happen to these grand, but slow-growing trees found only in parts of Africa. There's an effort to save trees from poachers and to establish commercial groves.

✿ None noted, but if you can grow it, you'll help keep the tree from extinction.

❀ The bark, leaves, fruit, and root.

♉ Most commonly used by the millions of men, worldwide, who suffer from an enlarged prostate and urinary problems that accompany that condition. Pygeum has also been used for the treatment of allergies, inflammation, kidney disease, digestive problems, fever, and even malaria. It is also believed that the herb is mildly antibiotic.

♦♦♦ Pygeum has been used to treat male pattern baldness.

🍽 None noted, except that the fruit is edible.

☞ Often found available with saw palmetto or by itself in capsule form. Purchase from a reputable source who is concerned about the decimation of this valuable tree.

📖 None noted, but what has happened to the tree is certainly a reminder to us that God has made us stewards of this planet and we have a great responsibility to take care of it.

❗ In large amounts could upset the stomach.

Rosemary

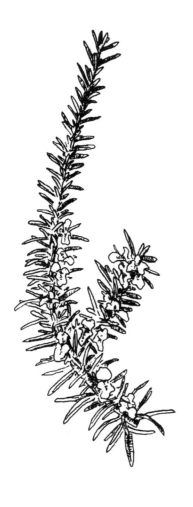

⚜ This evergreen plant grows like a tree and originally came from the Mediterranean. It has ash-colored bark and thick leathery leaves. It blooms a lovely and aromatic pale-blue flower in spring or early summer.

☼ I love to grow rosemary in the garden because of the aroma and the bright, shiny leaves. But if you live where the winters are substantial, you will want to bring it inside during those months. Rosemary will grow well in a pot. You will also find that it grows slowly and is managed best as a shrub.

🌿 Leaves and flowers.

♉ Like most culinary herbs, it's good for the digestion, and it's also said to be good for the liver. It's said that rosemary may raise blood pressure and help to improve circulation. This is a very powerful herb, as is true of most evergreens; so careful use is important.

⚕ Can be used to treat skin problems, bruises, and wounds. Rosemary is used more and more these days in the bathroom. I am seeing commercially-produced products like mouthwash and shampoo containing rosemary. I have oily hair, so I use a shampoo with rosemary in it, to help really clean my hair. The oil or a decoction of the leaves is used to treat sores, eczema, and bruises. As a scalp wash, it may help prevent baldness, because of its astringent properties.

🍽 A great culinary herb that adds flavor to any food.

☞ Boil ½ cup water and pour over 1 teaspoon of the flowers or leaves, and steep. Use a few dried leaves for seasoning.

📖 While not specifically mentioned in the Bible, there is a legend that says that it takes a rosemary plant 33 years to mature, the same length of Jesus' earthly life, and that in honor of him the plant never grows taller than a man's height. The Bible tells us, "Let everything that has breath praise the Lord!" (Ps. 150:6). I believe that every created thing reveals something about God, so maybe the legend of the rosemary has some truth to it.

❗ Use sparingly. A little goes a long way, and too much is considered poisonous.

Rue

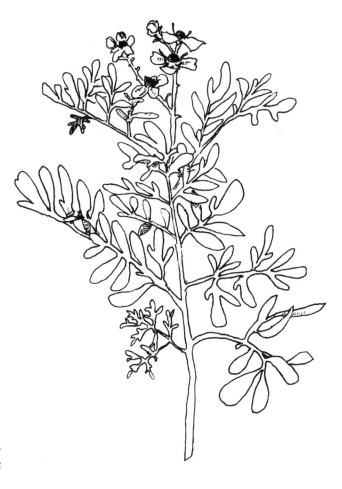

❂ Rue is an aromatic plant (although I find the smell distasteful). Once I grew some rue next to lavender, and it was a competition of smells. I eventually pulled the rue. It is a perennial that has its origin in the Bible lands. The plant grows to 3 feet and produces pretty, yellow blossoms in summer.

☼ The plant grows easily and is hardy; but it will quickly get out of hand and spread everywhere. If you are going to grow it, you may do well to plant it in a pot.

🌿 The whole plant.

⚱ Don't "rue the day." Considered a bitter herb, but in small amounts it's said to be good for the stomach, rheumatism, gout, and sciatic pain.

🏥 Salves are made from this herb to treat gout, rheumatism, and sciatica. Rue is also used as a medicine for the treatment of cattle and poultry. Rue is a very strong herb, so caution is important.

🍽 I'm certainly not suggesting any. But in olden days it was used to season food.

☞ For internal uses, steep 1 teaspoon herb per 1 cup water. For external uses, soak dried herb in water, then apply. Personally, I'd only use it externally.

📖 Mentioned in Luke 11:42 as one of the tithing herbs, so it was considered of value during Jesus' time. Rue and repentance walk hand in hand, and the plant is often called the "herb of grace" because of the grace Christ gives us after we truly rue our sinful ways and repent.

❗ Rue is considered poisonous with high use.

Sage

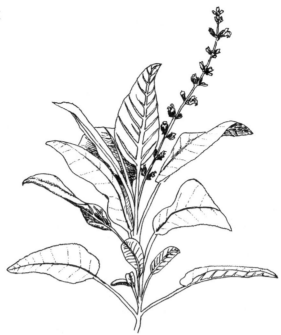

⚜ A perennial evergreen shrub with a woolly appearance and numerous varieties. Grows 1 to 2 feet tall. In the heart of the summer it produces flowers of purple, blue, or white.

✿ Grows well from seed and propagates from cuttings. Will grow as an annual in harsh climates, so you may want to keep this one confined to a pot, depending on your location.

🌿 The leaves.

🍵 Sage is said to help with nervous conditions, such as trembling, depression, and vertigo. It also helps the digestive system and the conditions of diarrhea and gastritis. It is used for respiratory conditions, as well.

🏥 As a gargle, sage tea is said to be good for sore throat, sore gums, laryngitis and tonsillitis. Leaves, finely crushed, are said to help relieve the pain and itching of insect bites.

🍲 This strong-smelling herb is great for the kitchen, combines well with other herbs, and it adds flavor to many dishes, especially poultry. I'm not sure a turkey dinner would be complete without sage as an ingredient. And do you notice that after a turkey dinner, you feel more satisfied and at peace? Maybe it is a combination of the turkey, which is also supposed to have a calming effect, and the sage seasoning. I like one variety called pineapple sage that has a distinctive, sweet scent and is milder, and tastes good in herbal sun teas and salads.

☞ Picking leaves before the plant flowers, steep 1 teaspoon in ½ cup water.

❗ This is a strong herb, so be careful. Extended use or excessive amounts are considered poisonous.

Savory

Winter Savory   Summer Savory

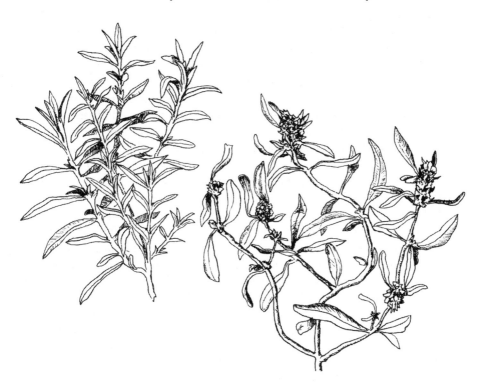

⚜ Savory originated in the Mediterranean. This plant is very flavorful and aromatic, especially the summer variety that grows as an annual. It grows to 1½ feet tall and produces small, pink-and-white flowers from mid-summer to early fall.

☼ Savory grows well in most conditions, but summer savory has a pretty short life, while winter savory in protected conditions can winter over. As your summer savory plant begins to bloom, pull off flowers to extend life.

🌹 The whole herb.

℧ The herb is good for a multitude of stomach concerns, especially if you drink it as a tea.

👬 Savory can also be used as a gargle for sore throat.

🍽 Cut it fresh into summertime salads or dry it for later use in soups and stews. This is a wonderful culinary herb with many uses and a great flavor. I like savory best in stews, soups, and other hot dishes.

Saw Palmetto

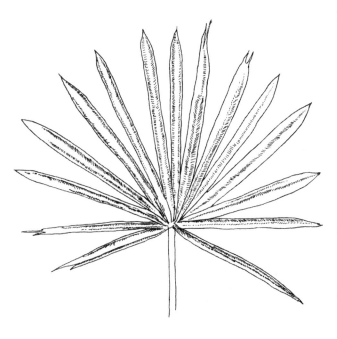

🌼 If you are a male and have reached your middle years and find yourself getting up in the night numerous times to urinate, then this herb may help you. I take it on a regular basis. The saw palmetto plant is found on the eastern seaboard in North Carolina, Georgia, and Florida. The tree grows to 20 feet tall. The fan-shaped, palm-like leaves and dark berries make this a distinctive plant. The berries grow in clusters, ripening in the fall.

✿ To plant saw palmetto outdoors, you will need to live in the south. But if you live in the north, you may be able to grow the tree in a pot and take it inside during harsh weather.

🌿 The berries.

🝾 Saw palmetto is being used and highly touted for the treatment of BPE or benign prostate enlargement. It helps to relax and tone the urinary tract, making urination easier throughout the day and helping you to not have to get up so often in the night. Many men, but not all, find this herb helpful. If you are a man experiencing these problems, then you need to see your doctor **now**! Prostate cancer is a major killer of older men.

But the palmetto herb is also good for other purposes. It's a good all-around body tonic, is said to help with symptoms of colds, asthma, and bronchitis. If you have had an extended illness, then it's said that palmetto can help rebuild your strength.

☞ Simmer 1 teaspoon dried berries in 1 cup water. The commercial production of this herb is excellent, and I prefer to buy capsules. But check the contents to be sure you are getting the maximum amount for your dollar. You will also find saw palmetto now as an additive in herbal teas and other products.

❗ Don't expect this herb to completely cure your prostate problems. It probably won't. Lifestyle change away from sedentary habits and high fat diet will make the biggest difference.

116

Skullcap
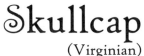
(Virginian)

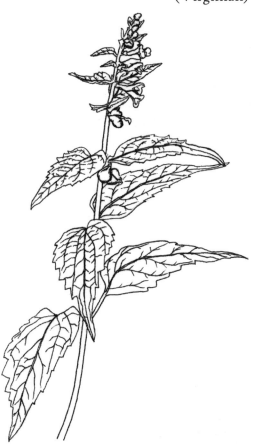

A perennial plant, *Scutellaria lateriflora*, common to northeastern America and Canada. The strange name comes from the description of what the flower looks like—a skullcap or a helmet. In fact skullcap is often called "helmet flower." It is also called "mad dog weed" because it was an early treatment for people who contracted the deadly rabies. The plant grows wild in wet areas, 1 to 3 feet tall with a yellow rootstock, and has small purple to blue flowers that bloom the length of summer.

This wild plant can be tamed for the garden. A perennial, it prefers sun and rich, damp soil. However, it has a short life and may be gone after a few years.

The whole plant, dried and ground into a powder.

Skullcap has been rediscovered as a headache medicine and a treatment for stress of which stress headaches are the symptom. Skullcap is helpful for related problems of nervousness and insomnia. It has also been used to treat people suffering from alcoholism or drug addiction in that skullcap helps with the withdrawals from addiction and alcohol poisoning. It is also suggested that skullcap is a good heart tonic, working in a way similar to hawthorn by strengthening the heart muscle. People suffering from muscle cramps, spasms, and pain have found relief with skullcap. Skullcap also helps some women dealing with menstruation pains. The list of nutrients that this plant has is impressive: calcium, iron, magnesium, manganese, phosphorus, potassium, selenium, zinc and vitamins B1, B2 and B3. This herb has a funny name but lots of benefits.

☞ In powder or in capsule form (preferred).

❗ Nothing specifically noted, but this is a strong herb, so only take the recommended dosage.

Slippery Elm

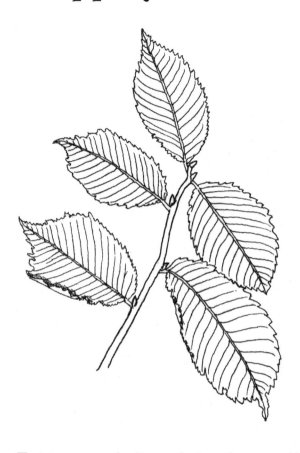

🌼 The name is certainly apropos. When your throat is so sore that every swallow is like being scraped by nails, drinking a cup of this wonderful herb makes it easier for needed fluids and food to go down. *Ulmus rubra* can be found growing in much of the U.S. and Canada. A deciduous tree that is smaller than its cousin, the common elm. The tree can grow to heights of 50 feet. It has a rough outer bark, oblong serrated leaves, and tiny flowers that grow in clusters and bloom in the early spring.

☼ Needs a good soil. Can be propagated by seeds or cuttings. Is highly suscepti-ble to Dutch elm disease.

🌿 The peeled-off inner bark, whitish in color and highly aromatic, turned into fine or coarse powder.

🗡 Most commonly, slippery elm is used to treat colds and sore throats. No matter how I try to keep from it, I seem to catch a couple of colds a year. Slippery elm tea certainly helps to relieve the sore throat, but don't stop there. Slippery elm is considered a safe and mild diuretic and also helps with urinary problems and complaints regarding gastric ulcers, colitis, and the bowels. This is a safe and natural way to combat the cold and flu season.

👪 The powder of the inner bark is also used as a suppository for female genitals and as an enema. The herb can be used as a poultice to treat skin irritations and inflammations.

🍽 The bark can be dried and ground to make into a flour and is said to be as nutritious and calming as oatmeal.

☞ Found in many homeopathic teas and in a powder. You can also peel the inner bark, which you will note has a slimy feel to it. This can be steeped in hot water for 15 minutes. A very safe herb.

Solomon's Seal

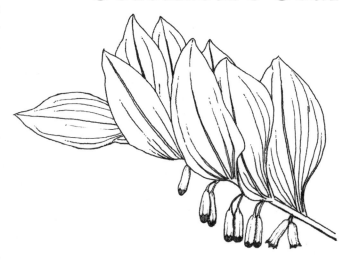

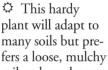 A perennial that grows mostly in the eastern U.S. and Canada. Reaches heights of only 1 to 2 feet. The upper half of the plant is leafy and droopy with bell-shaped flowers and an inedible, blue to black fruit looking like a blueberry.

☼ This hardy plant will adapt to many soils but prefers a loose, mulchy soil and regular watering. It will multiply pretty quickly by the underground root system. Can be started by seed propagation.

🌱 Rootstock.

☕ Native Americans have used this internally for centuries, but I do not recommend it. This plant is best used externally.

👥 Part of its name may come from what the plant does externally in treating bruises, bumps, scrapes and inflammations—It seals the wound. Solomon's seal is an astringent with cleansing and healing properties similar to aloe. It has also been used as a treatment for poison ivy. Ladies are using Solomon's seal again to help create a nicer complexion.

🍽 The young shoots, without the leaves, can be cooked like asparagus.

☞ The rootstock in powder for use as a poultice.

📖 The name may come from the rounded impressions on the rootstock which look like Hebrew letters formed when a seal is impressed in wax. The other possibility, and something for you to try with the flower of the plant, is to lightly dip it in ink or paint and press it onto paper. You should get something that looks like the Star of David which is also known as the Seal of Solomon. In the Song of Solomon 8:6, the writer says, "Place me like a seal over your heart, like a seal on your arm for love is as strong as death." Here the lover talks about how love is as strong as an unbreakable seal. We know that God's love for us is that strong. His love, purpose, authority and power are symbolically identified by his seal. God seals us with his Holy Spirit. When we become his, we receive the official mark that we are God's property and nobody can lay claim to us, including the devil. "Now it is God who ... anointed us, set his seal of ownership on us, and put his Spirit in our hearts" (Eph. 4:30). It's official. As a born-again believer, you are God's property forever and ever. May this plant remind you that you are sealed for good for God.

Soybean

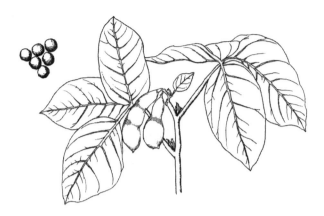

⊞ Certainly one of the best all-around vegetable/herbs. It offers nearly complete protein. High in antioxidants, isoflavones and fiber. Low in carbohydrates. No cholesterol or saturated fat. High in calcium, magnesium, lecithin, riboflavin, thiamin, folic acid, and iron. A legume native to eastern Asia where it has been the main dietary source for millenniums. Grows up to 3 feet like a bush bean, it flowers and then produces a pod. The bean can be harvested anytime from when the bean is green and immature until it is dried in the pod.

☼ Many varieties. Most need a warmer climate. Soybeans grow slowly, up to 120 days. For northern areas early season varieties are available, but soy cannot tolerate frost. It prefers a normal to sandy, somewhat alkaline soil and temperatures of 65-85° to germinate. The plant is highly susceptible to beetles, aphids, leafhoppers, blights, mildew and mold. Seeds start best when an inoculant is used to treat the seeds.

🐌 The bean (either green, mature, dried, or as soy nuts). A whole group of foods are made from soy: milk, tofu or bean curd, texturized meat substitutes, soy flour and pastas, soy butter and soy oil. People with lactose intolerance or diabetes may find soy products very helpful. Many consider soybean the perfect food. However, we live in a cursed world where nothing is perfect. A number of critics of soy indicate that soy may not be quite the miracle food that many tout.

⛉ The benefits seem nearly endless, from fighting colds to cancer. Soybean helps protect and build the bones and fight against osteoporosis, and protect against a number of cancers including breast cancer and prostate cancer. Also lowers the bad cholesterol, helps the cardio-vascular system, and relieves symptoms of menopause.

👫 Some Asians use tofu to promote healing of skin sores, lesions and ulcerations. There are more and more soy products for skin care on the market.

🍽 I like soy beans in their most natural and fresh green form ("edamame") picked right from the garden, cooked for 10-15 minutes and consumed with a little olive oil and light seasoning.

☞ Consume the bean in the many forms in which it is produced.

📖 None noted, however that doesn't minimize the fact that God created something absolutely wonderful when he made the simple soy.

❗ None noted although some people can be allergic to the bean and there are some critics who believe the bean does have some less than desirable effects.

Spikenard

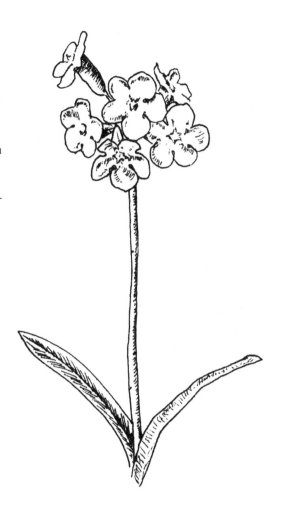

⊞ The spikenard of the Bible is probably not related to the spikenard available in North America. W. E. Shewell-Cooper suggests that the spikenard of the Bible is related to valerian and was exported from India. In America, "spikenard" refers to two varieties: *aralia racemosa* and *aralia nudicaulis*. Common names are: "Indian root," "life of man," "wild sarsaparilla," and "wild licorice." Found in rich woodland settings, American spikenard can grow to 6 feet, with roundish leaves and small greenish-white flowers that grow in umbels in the heat of summer.

☼ Prefers rich soil and partial shade. Grows wild in much of the country.

⚘ The rootstock.

⛉ The ground rootstock is used to treat respiratory conditions, including asthma. It is also said to have expectorant qualities. It is used in treating the symptoms of rheumatism and backaches.

⛊ The rootstock has been used topically to treat skin diseases, wounds, and inflammations.

⛐ It can be made into an aromatic and spicy-tasting tea.

☞ Steep 1 to 2 teaspoons ground rootstock per 1 cup water for tea. Pound the root into a poultice for external use.

📖 The spikenard of the Bible was a very costly substance. The root of the plant was used as a perfume and as an ointment, stored in alabaster boxes, and used for the anointing of special guests. The Song of Solomon mentions it as a perfume meant to arouse a person of the opposite sex. The lady love of this story is described as a garden where the heady fragrance of nard is present. (See Song 1:12, 4:13-14.) In the New Testament, Mary anointed Jesus with a complete container of nard. She poured it on his feet and wiped them with her hair. And the house was filled with the fragrance of the perfume. (See Jn. 12:3.) In this incredibly unselfish act, Mary shows herself as a true servant of the Lord. Are we willing to take on such a role of servanthood?

St. John's Wort

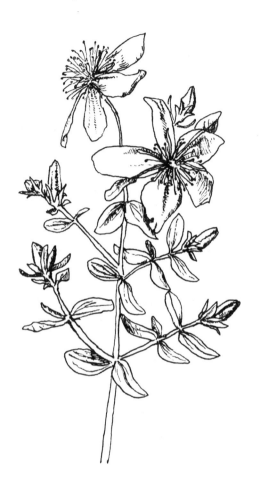

⊗ A lovely perennial with a funny name. Evergreen or a semi-evergreen, its leaves are shimmering green because of oil glands. The pretty flowers are yellow, 5-petaled, and bloom summer to early fall. Bears a fruit in the fall. The plant smells like turpentine. The word "wort" means "plant."

☼ Prefers warm, moist climate. It is utilized often as ground cover or hedge. Prefers part shade and likes adequate water.

✿ The entire above-ground plant.

✇ Currently very popular, but some medical authorities express concern. As a mood lifter and to treat mild depression, it's said to have a mild tranquilizing effect. People who suffer from anxiety and emotional upsets have been utilizing this as a way to even out the moods and avoid side effects from prescription drugs. Also considered a stomach aid. The flowers are said to be good for headaches, anemia, and insomnia. There is ongoing research being done on the herb's positive effect upon people suffering with HIV and AIDS.

⚕ The plant's oil is used for treating burns, wounds, sores, bruises, etc.

☞ A tea is made with 1 teaspoon dried leaves and flowers to ½ cup water. Oil is available. Because of the popularity of the herb, capsules, herb teas, etc. are readily available. Check labels to make sure you are getting the real thing.

📖 The name is steeped in mystery. It seems that the St. John referred to here is not St. John the Apostle, but John the Baptist, the great prophet who announced the coming of the Lord Jesus and who was eventually executed for his faith. Salome called for John's head and he died of decapitation by the sword. The name of the plant comes from the fact that when you take the leaves and squeeze them between your fingers, the plant exudes a reddish oil resembling blood.

❗ St. John's wort has come under fire because of its possible effects on people taking prescription drugs, so check with your doctor. Also, there may be an increase of sun sensitivity for people who take it regularly.

Sunflower

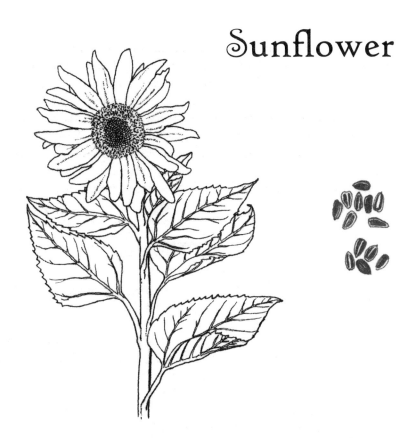

🌼 Sunflowers, *Helianthus annuus*, grow wild all across America. Dozens of varieties have been developed in many colors and sizes. Common sunflower is a native of Mexico and South America. Grown as an annual. In some warmer climates some varieties will grow as perennials. The plants range from a few feet tall to 15 feet. I grew one accidentally, or it grew itself with very little help from me, and it reached beyond the eaves of my house! The flowers can grow from as small as a few inches across to as much as 15 to 18 inches with hundreds of seeds. The common sunflower is that bright sun-yellow color, but there are many varieties of reds, magentas, blacks, etc. The heart-shaped leaf grows from a few inches to 12 inches long and 6 inches across. Jerusalem artichoke is also of the sunflower family. If you really like sunflowers, check out the National Sunflower Association online. They provide information and products.

☼ I love to grow these great beauties. They're relatively easy to start and grow fast. At the end of the season I take the big flower heads, dry them, separate out the seeds, roast them, and enjoy them for months. Sunflowers appreciate poor soil and will grow just about anywhere. But true to their name, the more sun they get, the taller and bigger they grow. You can start them directly in the ground, but you'll get a head start by starting them indoors or in a greenhouse. True summer-loving plants, they cannot tolerate even a hint of frost. If you're

(Sunflower continued on next page)

into "seedin' and spittin'," look for "Mammoth Russian" varieties. These are what the commercial growers market and baseball players love to chew and spit.

🌹 Seeds. But virtually all parts of the plant were originally used by people across the Americas and now across much of the world, and for different purposes. Many farmers and ranchers will feed the leaves to their stock. The fiber of the stalk can be used to make paper or even as fire kindling. Sunflower oil, with its high digestibility rates is nearly as good for you as olive oil. Even the flower petals can be used to extract a yellow dye.

🝙 The greatest value of the sunflower seed is as a simple and nutritious food. Sunflower seeds are mildly diuretic. For a tea that may help as an expectorant and to ease a cough caused by colds and other respiratory problems, steep the seeds, oil, or flower petals. People have even used the seeds, oil and petals to treat whooping cough. Sunflower seeds are high in vitamin E and polyunsaturates. The oil may help lower cholesterol.

👬 The oil is used in making lotions, soaps, and massage oils and perfumes for skin and hair. Wrapping sufferers of malaria in the leaves has been used to break the fever.

🍽 Native Americans used sunflower much like corn, grinding it into meal and flour. Steeping roasted nuts and shells can produce a coffee or tea substitute. We tend to eat sunflower seeds with too much salt, so try unsalted seeds in virtually anything you want. I think the health benefits will be better.

☞ The dry roasted seed. The seed compressed into an oil. The shell, seed, oil, and flower steeped as a tea.

📖 In a recent summer I planted sunflowers, but I was surprised to find them sprouting in places I had not planted them. One such plant grew to 12 feet before it developed a flower, while another grew such a thick stalk that the fully developed sunflower was 15 inches in diameter, with leaves similar in size. I marveled at the size of the plants and then began to study the leaves. I noticed that the leaves were in the perfect shape of the valentine heart we see in February.

Look at a sunflower leaf, large or small, and you will notice that from the stem three veins separate to make up the backbones of the leaves. The largest extends down the middle and the other two, left and right, extend to the middle of each half. In this I discovered a plant parable of the triune nature of God. Joined together and yet separated, each having a separate function. The last thing I noticed is that the edges of this botanical heart are scalloped; the edges almost resemble the edge of a saw blade. I wondered about that. Here is a picture of the love of God in the leaf, the shape of the heart. Here is another picture of God in three surrounded by the shape of love and yet here are the jagged edges of the outside of the leave. If you could imagine that this leaf were a saw blade and you were to rub your finger or hand across it you may find that it would cut and you would bleed. Here was a love that God-in-three gave us that was so sweet, so sacrificial, and yet so severe that blood would run to prove it.

I'll never look at a sunflower the same again. In fact I will find it hard to not spell it "Sonflower."

Tarragon
(French)

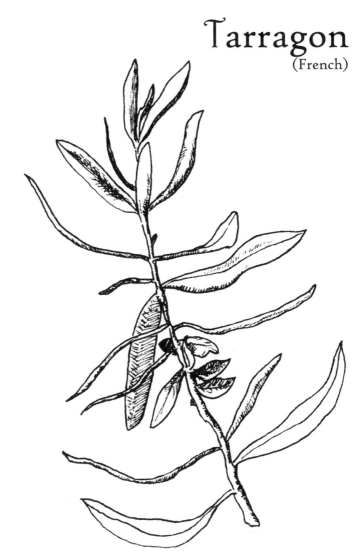

▣ Tarragon is another attractive plant for the garden or window sill. This is a perennial plant that usually is grown as an annual. Many varieties of this plant are now available. Tarragon has narrow, dark-green leaves and small, white-to-green or yellow flowers. The plant grows to 2 feet tall.

✿ Tarragon is easy enough to grow in the garden or in a pot, but the plant prefers a dry, warm setting, and well-drained, rich soil.

❀ The leaves.

🗡 A French chef's favorite, this herb is good for the digestive system and will help to settle the stomach and help the kidneys to function better. A tea of tarragon helps relieve insomnia.

♙♙ An infusion of the leaves is said to help relieve toothache, cuts and sores. It may act as a painkiller.

🍽 The plant has a slight licorice taste. It is often used in French cuisine and with seafood. For a little flair, try adding some taragon to the vinegar you use for seasoning.

☞ Make a tea of ½ teaspoon dried leaves to ½ cup water.

Tea

Red, White, Green

Wave the red, white and green for great health. Better yet, drink it. Here are three healthful, flavorful teas that contain an amazing amount of beneficial properties. Think about these the next time you go for a sugar-laden soft drink.

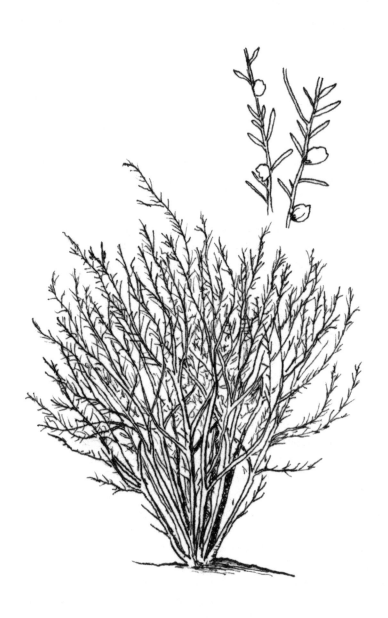

RED TEA (*ROOIBOS*) OR REDBUSH (Pictured at left)

▣ This semi-tropical plant is found in the dry mountainous areas of South Africa where it has been used as a beverage for centuries. In America, red tea is becoming very popular because of the high amount of antioxidants it contains. Plus it is a highly favorable tea. That plant is a shrub that grows to heights of no more than 6 feet. It has bright green, thin, straight leaves with small yellow flowers and pods. During the processing of the leaves, their color turns to a dark reddish brown, hence the name and the color of the tea.

☼ The plant is somewhat adaptable to colder weather and can endure short mild frosts. Prefers a dry, sandy soil.

❀ Leaves and roots.

℧ Rooibos is high in vitamin C and in antioxidants, so if you drink green tea for that purpose, you may like red tea as well. I love the flavor because it is stronger than the mild green tea and yet it contains no caffeine. Red tea may also help with soothing the symptoms of allergies.

✋ Much research is still being done on rooibos, but it is said that the leaves are good for treating eczema and other skin complaints.

🍲 Rooibos has been used to flavor sauces.

☞ Dry the leaves or the root stock for tea.

❗ Seems to be very safe. No concerns noted.

WHITE TEA

▣ I have included white tea because of its growing popularity. However, there is no difference between white, green or black tea because it comes from the same plant (see drawing next page). It's just a matter of the timing and the method of the processing. At one time, white tea was reserved for royalty or for the rich. To produce white tea, the leaves of the plant are harvested before they are fully opened, thus the immature, undeveloped leaves. This makes the amount of tea to be harvested much more scarce and expensive. White tea is considered more delicate and sweet in flavor and should be brewed in hot, but not boiling, water. There are some indications that white tea may have more antioxidants than green tea, but that is still open for debate. There are numerous varieties of this tea. Most are produced in China, Japan and, to a lesser degree, in India.

(Tea continued on next page)

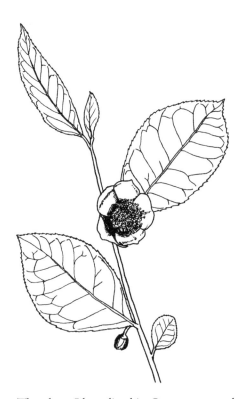

GREEN TEA
(*Camellia Sinensis*)

This herb is my favorite morning, noon and night hot or cold drink. The *Camellia Sinensis* is a small evergreen tree or shrub that reaches to 15 feet tall and is indigenous to eastern and southern Asia. Look for white and pink blooms and leathery leaves. At full height, leaves grow to 5 inches long and flowers to 1½ inches. This attractive plant is fun to have around. It's just finicky in its early years. I have grown them unsuccessfully for the past few years. The plant, however, is readily available these days from nurseries, so you can grow your own tea. Hundreds of varieties.

Makes a good container plant. Very tender perennial. Will not tolerate even a hint of frost, arid conditions, or hot sun. Needs partial shade. The places I have lived in Oregon are too harsh for this plant to weather out the year.

Leaves.

I started drinking this tea, the decaffeinated version, because of a little bladder infection that was plaguing me. Green tea chased it away in a day or so. And I have been hooked ever since, now drinking a few cups daily. Usually it is how I begin my day and often it is how I end it. The tea companies should owe me stock for being such a good customer! Green tea comes from the same plant that black tea comes from. It is the processing that makes the difference. Green tea is also a powerful antioxidant and cancer fighter. The tea helps to lower dangerous cholesterol levels, stimulates the immune system, fights tooth decay, helps to regulate blood sugars, combats mental fatigue, and may help with weight regulation and benign prostate enlargement. No wonder I feel so good!!

Green tea extract is being used in lotions and such for the skin, so look for these products.

Green tea has a very satisfying flavor that keeps you looking forward to it and coming back. It makes a great iced tea for hot days; very refreshing, especially with a sprig of mint added. Green tea is often what you get as part of your dinner at your favorite Asian restaurant.

Dry the leaves and make into a tea.

If you have problems with caffeine, like I do, then stick with the decaf varieties that are readily available.

Tea Tree

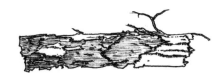

▣ Incorrectly named, the tea tree, *Melaleuca alternifolia* or *Melaleuca leucadendron*, is not to be confused with *Camellia sinensis*, from which we get white, green and black tea. In fact the oil from tea tree should not be consumed internally (see below). Tea tree oil is also sometimes known as "Cajuput." The tea tree oil that you would purchase today is more likely to come from *Melaleuca alternifolia*, which is a tender evergreen found in Australian swampy areas and discovered for European and American use by the famed explorer Captain Cook. The tree has a slim trunk, long leathery leaves, and small flowers. It is aromatically pungent.

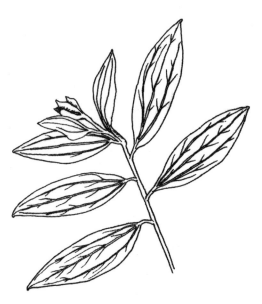

☼ This is a tropical plant. It can be grown from cuttings. However, there are a number of varieties of this tree, and one that has been cultivated for the states with warmer climates is *Leptospermum laevigatum*.

🌿 Leaves and the extracted essential oil that comes from them. Often mixed with vegetable, vitamin, or other herbal oils.

☕ None suggested. Toxic.

🏃 Tea tree oil may be one of the best and most wonderful natural ways to treat the skin. Tea tree oil has strong disinfectant qualities and is a great germicide. It is a great way to clean the skin after a wound, and it is so effective that people have found healing for a myriad of skin complaints from acne or ringworm to fungal problems like athlete's foot. It helps with hair and scalp complaints, including head lice. Tea tree oil will soothe insect bites, help with scabies, warts, and even outbreaks of herpes. Tea tree oil is used—carefully, because you don't want to swallow it!—as a gargle for colds, mouth and gum ailments, and diseased and sore throats. It is also an effective feminine douche and is often effective against yeast infections. The oil is very pungent and everyone will know you are using it!

☞ The oil is readily available in health food and herbal stores. Follow the directions provided by the supplier.

❗ This is a strong oil and if it causes skin irritation, discontinue. The oil should absolutely not be swallowed.

Thyme

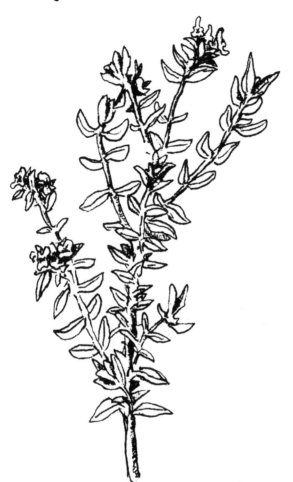

🏵 This is another great culinary herb that grows well in the garden or year-round in a window box. A small perennial with prolific, but small leaves and small, blue-to-purple flowers that bloom late spring to late summer, depending upon the variety and climate. Thyme rarely grows taller than 1 foot. You will notice a heady aroma, especially in the heat of the day. There are a number of varieties of this plant, including Mother of Thyme, Creeping Thyme, Lemon Thyme, etc.

☼ This plant grows easily and is quite hardy. It also makes a good ground cover that doesn't spread too rapidly. A nice addition to the flower garden, as well as the herb garden.

🌹 The whole plant.

℧ Thyme is a good and mild herb that works well as an all-around digestive aid. It is also said to help with respiratory conditions in clearing up congestion. Women may find it helpful during the menstrual cycle.

👪 Add thyme to your bath. It is said to be stimulating to the system and to reduce nervousness. Thyme is also used externally to treat tumors, wounds, bruises, and rheumatism.

🍽 Many uses in the kitchen. I like to pick thyme leaves to add not only to cooked Italian dishes, but fresh salsas and salads.

☞ Fresh or dried leaves for culinary uses or to make a tea. Use 1 or 2 teaspoons of leaves to 1 cup of boiling water. Thyme oil is also available.

Uva Ursi

Bearberry

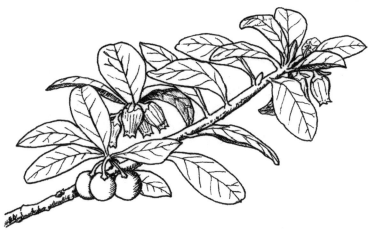

⊞ This plant is native to the Northern Hemisphere and it has a number of names, the most common being bearberry, kinnikinnick and Upland cranberry. Bearberry is a low-growing, creeping plant found in many forest areas. Uva ursi is related to manzanita, azalea, and rhododendron, which grow in abundance in my part of the world. It has spoon-shaped, leathery leaves, red woody branches, small delicate white and pink flowers, and bright red berries. Native Americans used the berry for food and the leaves as one of the ingredients in a combination of plants to be used for smoking. However, the herb has much better uses than that.

✿ Uva ursi prefers a dry, sandy or gravelly soil and has been cultivated as an effective, drought-tolerant ground cover.

🌹 Leaves and berries.

🗘 This indigenous plant is being rediscovered for a number of wonderful healing properties, because it is high in tannins. It is being used as a bacteria fighter and as a heart tonic similar to hawthorn in that it can help with high blood pressure. It is considered a tonic for the weakened heart. It has also been used for disorders of the liver, pancreas, spleen, and small intestine. It is a diuretic and its best use may be for kidney, bladder, and urinary tract infections, and it may help treat kidney stones. The herb is being used by men for prostate problems. Women have used uva ursi for a number of female complaints. It is even being used to treat diabetes.

👬 Uva ursi has been used as a topical to treat skin wounds.

🍴 The berries, cooked, have a pleasant taste, but a mealy texture.

☞ Leaves are collected in the fall and dried in thin loose layers. For a topical to the skin, use dried crushed leaves. For your safety, if you are going to take it internally, purchase uva ursi products at your favorite health food store.

❗ This is a strong herb considered toxic if over used. It should not be used by pregnant or nursing women, or by children.

Valerian

(Fragrant)

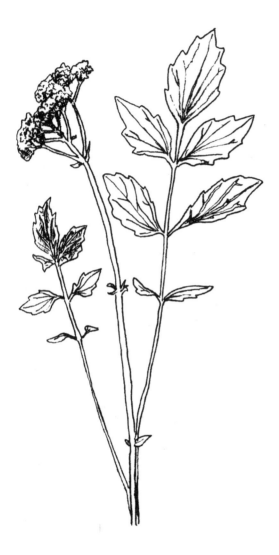

⊞ Whoever termed this herb "fragrant" doesn't have the same olfactory senses that I have. If I were to give it a name, I would call it "stinky valerian." But don't let the smell chase you off. This herb has benefits. The perennial plant grows up to 4 feet tall and is found in the eastern half of North America. The plant has a long stem, pinnate leaves that stay close to the ground, and small, fragrant flowers of red to white color that bloom in the heart of summer.

☼ The hardy plant can handle sun or shade. It is good for the back of flower beds. But it will encroach on other plants.

🌱 The root.

♉ This plant is currently touted as an alternative to valium and other powerful prescription sedatives. People use it for nervousness and for treating panic attack syndromes. It is considered a much safer alternative to prescription drugs; but check with your doctor. It certainly should not be taken in concert with these kinds of prescribed medicines. Valerian is also said to help with insomnia, migraine headaches, muscle cramping, menstrual symptoms, and PMS.

♈ Valerian is used externally to treat skin sores and acne.

☞ The rootstock is boiled. Suggested use is 2 teaspoons per pint of water. Capsules are also available and easier to take because of the unpleasant smell and taste of valerian root.

❢ Large amounts of valerian are considered poisonous in that they can cause paralysis and may adversely affect the heart. Do not take valerian in addition to medication for insomnia or anxiety.

Violet

(Garden, Sweet, Wild)

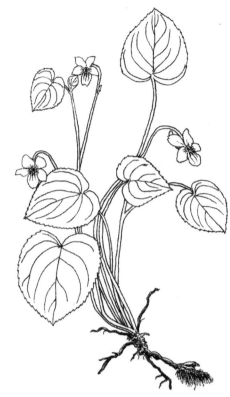

⊞ I love violets! For a person who would like to garden year around but can't because of the climate I live in, violets are a reminder and a precursor to me of months of gardening enjoyment coming up. Violets are one of the few hardy perennials that manage to grow and sometimes bloom even in the snow. There are over 300 varieties of this plant and, I suppose, more being cultivated all the time. This is also a plant that grows in the wild in many places, so you can utilize them from the garden or from the wild.

☼ Hardy. Grows everywhere but doesn't tolerate hot weather with constant sun. Most varieties prefer cooler weather, rich soil and require partial shade to thrive. Violets spread from the underground root system and seeds. I am amazed at all the places I find them sprouting up where I never planted them, including the grassy sections of my yard.

🏵 The whole plant. Flowers, leaves and rootstock.

� The plant has a number of useful properties, but it seems to shine for respiratory complaints. The leaves can be used in a tea as a throat gargle and for headaches. The root is good as an expectorant. The flowers and rootstock, in a tea, will help with colds and coughs. Violet is considered a calmative, so people have used it for everything from insomnia to hysteria. Violet can also be used as a mild laxative.

🏥 Used to treat chronic skin conditions such as eczema. Can be used for a number of skin eruptions, and for muscle, tension, head, and neck aches.

🍽 Considered a good source of vitamin C. Stems, leaves and flowers make a quick and colorful addition to a salad. You can also cook the greens as you would spinach. Dry the leaves for a pleasant tea. Violet can be cooked into breads, cookies, jams and jellies. And if you like to make herbal-scented vinegar, try using violets.

☞ For medicinal purposes, this plant is best used as a tea or a syrup by soaking and then boiling in water.

❗ Some varieties can be stronger than others and could cause an upset stomach, vomiting, and/or diarrhea if over-used.

Walnut

Black Walnut

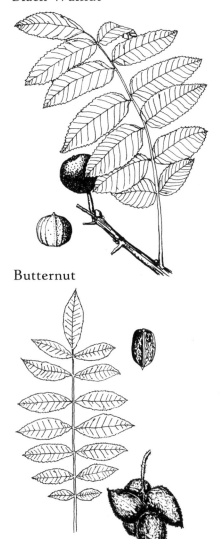

Butternut

🔲 Two varieties of walnut trees are found in North America that produce the common walnut.

☼ Grows in temperate climates almost anywhere. Make sure you have enough space if you plan to grow a walnut tree in your backyard, because it will grow 40 to 60 feet tall. Will provide a lot of shade. Some can live to 300 years, so it will outlast you and probably your house.

🌿 Black walnut: bark, leaves, and fruit. Butternut: the bark.

🗡 My research indicated many uses. I have listed the most common ones, but this wonderful tree deserves your investigation. Black walnut bark, infused as a tea, helps to relieve constipation and bacterial and parasitic infections. Also said to be good as mouthwash for mouth sores and inflamed tonsils. Infusions of butternut bark is said to be an effective, soothing laxative for people who have chronic problems with constipation. Drinking it may also help with colds, fevers, and flu. Of course, both of these nuts, or fruits, are edible. Nuts may be a superior substitute for meat; and they are cholesterol fighters.

👭 Because of its astringent properties, the leaves of the black walnut can be used for cleaning and washing of skin and to treat warts, eczema, herpes, psoriasis, and ringworm.

🍽 Many. See recipe section for some wonderful treats utilizing nuts.

☞ 1 teaspoon bark tea per 1 cup water.

📖 Solomon wrote, "I went down to the grove of nut trees to look at the new growth in the valley" (Song 6:11a). He must have had quite the garden, including this great tree. Isn't it wonderful, God gives us so much in one tree: shade, beauty, health-giving food. And any furniture maker will tell you that walnut furniture is not only pretty, but because of its hardness and durability, will be in use for generations.

❗ Before you peel bark from your tree to make tea, check with your local herbalist for best options.

Wild Oregon Grape

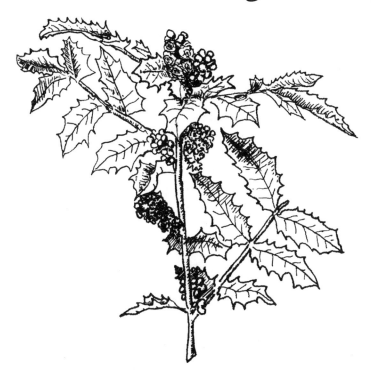

🏵 This plant is found in my neck of the woods (Oregon); but it grows wild from Northern California to British Columbia, and east to Idaho. I think this is a very pretty plant, with it shiny, leather-like leaves, yellow flowers that bloom in spring, and blue berries. The plant can exceed 6 feet in height. It is hardy and grows almost anywhere, but seems to prefer a dryer climate.

✿ Wild Oregon grape can be grown in a pot or as an ornamental in the garden. The birds will appreciate the berries.

🌿 The root and the berries.

🝙 This herb has antiseptic qualities and is considered a diuretic. It also has laxative qualities. It has been touted as a blood purifier and helpful for lowering blood pressure. It is also said to be a tonic for the liver and the spleen.

👬 Utilizing a tincture, it is said the herb helps with skin conditions such as acne, eczema, and psoriasis.

🍽 I have not tried it. I hear that the berries make a nice jam.

☞ Utilizing the root in its second year, 1 teaspoon herb to 1 cup water.

❗ It is suggested that people with existing liver conditions not use wild Oregon grape without consulting their doctor. This is a powerful herb, so conscientious use is necessary.

Wild Yam

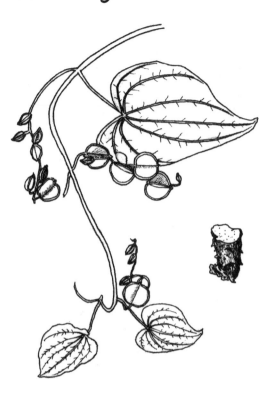

🦑 Wild yam is found in much of the U.S., but mostly from the Midwest to the Eastern Seaboard and down in to the Southeast. In some parts of the country it is considered a noxious weed. Wild yam is known by many different names and has over 800 species. A vine, it grows as an annual, and looks similar to ivy. The vine can grow to lengths of up to 18 feet long with leaves 2 to 6 inches long and green to yellow flowers that bloom late spring to early summer. The species that is being cultivated the most for its herbal benefits is "wild Mexican yam."

☼ Available through herbal seed growers. Can be planted by seed or root division. Prefers plenty of sun and rich soil. Harvest time comes in the fall when the tuber or rhizome is mature.

🌿 Root and rhizome.

☝ Wild yam has been used commercially in the production of contraceptives, topical hormones, and steroid drugs that are pretty much ineffective. There has been much controversy about these uses of the herb, and most professionals will caution you about use of wild yam for the above-mentioned purposes.

Best and safest use seems to be for the treatment of pain and inflammation because of the phytosterols, alkaloids and tannins found in this plant. This age-old traditional remedy utilized first by the natives has become very popular natural treatment for muscle pain and cramps, arthritis, rheumatism, neuralgia and for women's menstrual and post-menstrual complaints. It is used more and more by women desiring natural childbirth with less pain. Wild yam, because of these relaxing properties, may be helpful for an array of digestive complaints including the gall bladder, diverticulitis, and irritable bowel syndrome.

👪 Wild yam topicals, such as creams, are available.

🍽 It is considered edible, although it tastes from bland to bitter.

☞ The root or tuber is dried and made into a tea. Capsules are also available.

❗ There's a lot of hype out there about wild yam as some sort of miracle herb that will do a whole lot more than it is meant to do, so be careful about your reasons for utilizing it. This is a relatively safe herb when used for its proper healing qualities and in proper dosages.

Wintergreen

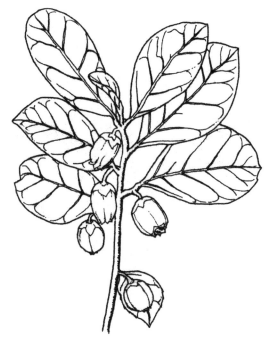

⌬ A delightful plant to grow on the shady side of the garden. A native to America, specifically *Gaultheria procumbens* on the east coast. In the west we have *Gaultheria ovatifolia* which is quite similar. A small, shrubby evergreen plant, with dark-green shiny leaves, the plant grows to less than a foot tall and is often found under such plants as rhododendrons. Wintergreen has droopy white flowers in the spring followed by bright red berries. Makes a great ground cover for a shady damp area. If you haven't tasted true wintergreen flavor, then you'll find the berries have a unique, if even peculiar, but pleasant taste. The leaves, dried and steeped in a tea, have the same taste.

☼ Wintergreen plants are available at nurseries. Similar in disposition to rhododendron and azalea, wintergreen likes a damp soil, somewhat acidic and with partial shade. Treat it as an under-story plant by providing it with that kind of microclimate. I have mine planted on the north side of the house. The plant can be divided at the root suckers and the seeds from the berries can be propagated.

🌹 Leaves and berries and the essential oil.

🗘 Wintergreen tea has been used for centuries by Native Americans as an effective treatment for sore muscles and aching joints, and for good reason. The leaves contain methyl salicylate which is similar to aspirin, and so you might find that it chases off a headache and relieves some of the discomfort of a toothache. Wintergreen is also said to be good as a tonic for the circulatory system. It may even help with urinary problems, gas, and other digestive disorders.

⚘ The leaves are used in a poultice or diluted oil, topically for skin complaints as well as aches and pains.

🍽 The leaves and berries steeped for tea. New tender leaves in a salad. For something really unique, try sampling a ripe red berry. You will notice a very distinct and sweet flavor. My first thought was, "This doesn't taste like wintergreen." That is because the gums, mints and such that they say have a wintergreen flavor, don't.

☞ The leaves or berries as a poultice or diluted oil.

❗ Wintergreen seems to be a very safe herb, but the oil must be diluted if used topically otherwise it may irritate the skin.

Witch Hazel

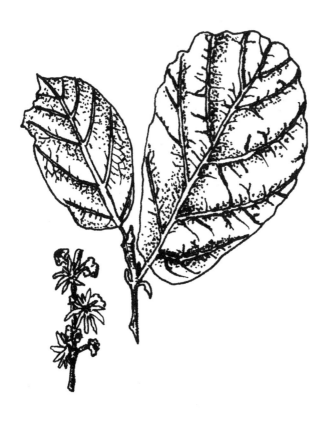

⬛ This deciduous little tree grows in the eastern half of North America, as far as the midwest. The tree can grow to 15 feet tall. It has eliptical leaves and blossoms of fragrant, yellow flowers. It blooms in autumn, when the leaves change to yellow and drop. The name is steeped in folklore that is hard to trace. In the early days of America, the tree branches were used as divining rods. There seems to be a root to the name that may mean "wican" which would have occultic roots. Many herbs were and are used in potions, etc., by people who worship and practice the occult. The reality is that what God has made for good is sometimes used for evil.

☼ The witch hazel plant grows in most zones. It needs moderate water and can handle sun or shade.

🌱 Leaves and bark.

⚗ Witch hazel was readily available in Grandma's medicine cabinet 50 years ago; and it still has great uses today. Witch hazel is used predominately for its astringent or cleansing properties, internally and externally. It is used internally as a gargle for mouth and throat irritations, and as a cure for diarrhea.

👫 A skin tonic. Witch hazel is used for an assortment of skin irritations and disorders, such as bruises, insect bites and stings, minor burns, vaginal irritations, and hemorrhoids.

☞ For a tea, utilize 1 teaspoon bark or leaves to 1 cup boiling water, and infuse for 10 to 15 minutes. You may purchase the distillate and extract in liquid form, available at pharmacies, herb shops, and natural food stores.

Wormwood

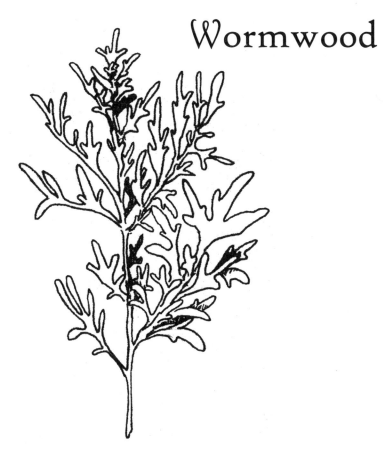

🌼 A perennial plant with a soft, silky appearance that grows in much of the United States, and is also found in the Bible lands. This is the main source of a substance called absinthe which is very dangerous. Wormwood has a strong, pungent and somewhat unpleasant odor. It has a very bitter taste, hence the name. The plant has silvery-gray leaves and small, yellow flowers. It grows to 4 feet tall.

✿ Wormwood makes an interesting addition to the garden and grows easily enough, but it will encroach on other plants. It is a strong herb and seems to have a negative effect upon other, more delicate annuals in the garden. I have noticed, while working with this plant, an almost toxic effect upon my skin.

🌿 Leaves and flowering tops.

🝙 GREAT CAUTION must be exercised in utilizing this plant. Wormwood is used as a stomach tonic, helping with digestion, gas, and lack of appetite. It may help with heartburn, and it is strong enough to expel intestinal worms. It is also said to help to stimulate the liver and the gall bladder.

👬 Wormwood oil acts as an anesthetic and helps relieve pain associated with rheumatism and arthritis. You may find that this herb enclosed in a sachet may keep the moths away from the clothes in your closet.

(Wormwood continued on next page)

☞ Herb specialist John Lust suggests steeping 2 teaspoons of leaves and tops in 1 cup of water; then take by the teaspoonful, ½ cup per day.

📖 Wormwood is mentioned numerous times in the Bible and always in reference to calamity and bitter experiences. Deuteronomy 29:18 describes turning from the Lord, idolatry and worshipping other gods as a bitter root that leads to a bitter poison. In Proverbs 5:4 adultery is described as an act that leads to death with reference to the bitterness associated with wormwood and the results thereof. Amos 5:7 compares unrepentance to bitter wormwood. And certainly in the last days, the tribulation and the judgment of God toward humankind on this earth will compare with the bitterness of wormwood. Revelation 8:10-11 speaks of this horrific time: "The third angel sounded his trumpet, and a great star, blazing like a torch, fell from the sky on a third of the rivers and on the springs of water—the name of the star is Wormwood. A third of the waters turned bitter, and many people died from the waters that had become bitter."

God makes clear to us that our choice to be disobedient and turn away from him will be a bitter choice with eternal consequences. I can't help thinking of those who have used this earth—and the gifts that God has given them—for their own selfish desires. Whether we like it or not—even understand it or not—God is a jealous God. Those who turn away from him and choose to worship other things will pay bitterly for their choice. Those who have taken the herbs with their wonderful properties which have been given to us by God, and used them in practices of the occult, will face a bitter end. The prophet Jeremiah saw himself and humankind for what they really are: sinful and disobedient. He says that "God has filled me with bitter herbs [wormwood]" (Lam. 3:15). Jeremiah knows that it is his willingness to repent and turn to the Lord that "breaks the spell" of the judgment he faces and that we all face. "Yet I call this to mind," he says, "and therefore I have hope: Because of the Lord's great love we are not consumed, for his compassions never fail. They are new every morning; great is your faithfulness" (Lam. 3:21-23).

How is your relationship with God? Have you accepted the forgiveness and the grace of Jesus Christ who was nailed to a bloody cross? Our sins are forgivable; and a new day starts for us when we are willing to turn away from sin and turn back to the One who created us, loves us, and wants us with him for eternity. May wormwood always be a reminder of the bitterness of a life—or an eternity—without God.

❗ The oil of wormwood is called absinthe, and was once used in making alcoholic beverages, but has been banned because it is poisonous. People have died from it. I would not use wormwood without seeking advice from knowledgeable and reliable medical authorities.

Yellow Dock

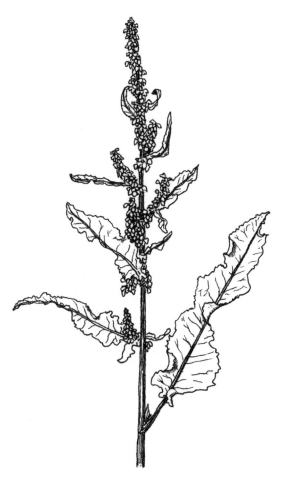

⊛ Similar to and related to rhubarb and sorrel, this roadside weed is found in much of the U.S. and many consider it a nuisance because is grows abundantly. It gets part of its name from the color of the root which is yellow and grows to a foot in length and up to an inch thick. It is the root that is sought for its medicinal purposes. The plant can grow to 3 feet tall with oblong, pale-green leaves and bushy brownish green flowers, and it produces a small fruit or nut.

☼ No recommendations. It grows everywhere and you would probably yank it out of your yard if you found more than one.

🌺 Specifically the root but also the leaves.

🍵 Yellow dock has astringent and purgative qualities and is considered a whole body tonic. It is said to have good effects upon the liver, gall bladder, gastric and vascular system. Yellow dock has been considered a blood purifier for centuries.

👪 Yellow dock makes a great topical ointment for the skin when itching, sores, swelling, and scabbing are needing treatment. Native Americans would use the boiled leaves as a poultice to treat boils and such. In fact, yellow dock is enjoying a new popularity because of its benefits for the skin. You can find yellow dock ointments and such at your health food store.

🍽 Not recommended. The fresh tender leaves have been consumed, but they have a mild laxative effect. And there is new concern that because the leaves contain oxalates that they may cause oxalic acid poisoning.

☞ The root is boiled and can be taken internally or pulverized into a powder for topical treatments.

❗ The leaves are not for culinary consumption. This is a strong herb, so only take as directed.

Yerba Santa

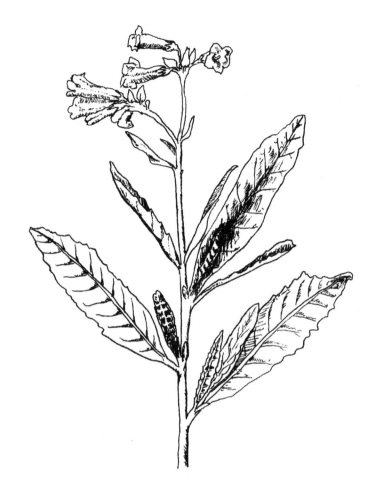

❊ This herb is a native to the west where I live and it can be found in Oregon and California. It is an aromatic plant that can grow to 7 feet tall. It has dark, leathery leaves and white- to lavender-colored flowers that bloom late spring to mid summer.

☼ Prefers a dryer climate.

❧ The leaves.

♆ Introduced to early European Americans by the Native Americans. It was used as a treatment for bronchial congestion, hay fever, asthma, and even tuberculosis. Yerba santa was also used as an alternative for tobacco.

⚕ A poultice can be made from the leaves for treating skin inflammations, injuries, bruises, sprains, wounds, and insect bites.

☞ 1 teaspoon of leaves to 1 cup of water.

Yucca

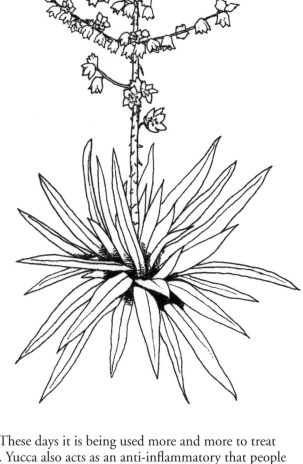

❁ A perennial evergreen with numerous species and found growing in much of the U.S., but predominantly in arid and desert areas. This plant, specifically *Yucca baccata* pictured here, was a mainstay herb and food source for the natives for millenniums. Yucca has tough sword-like leaves. I especially like the flowering creamy-white blooms of this plant.

☼ If you live in the northern areas like I do, then keeping a yucca would be the same as keeping a cactus that you would grow in a pot and take out during the warm months. I have a Joshua tree that I have been growing for years that is part of this huge family of plants commonly called yucca.

🌿 Pretty much the whole plant.

↯ Yucca is considered a blood tonic or purifier. These days it is being used more and more to treat arthritis and osteoporosis. Yucca also acts as an anti-inflammatory that people utilize for sore backs and muscles.

🎎 Yucca is being used more and more for hair treatment in shampoos and conditioners because of its astringent properties similar to aloe.

🍽 Native Americans consume the fruits. They are high in vitamins B, beta-carotene, calcium, iron, magnesium, and zinc.

☞ You can use fresh-cut yucca, one cup of the leaves to 2 cups of water, but it is also available in capsule form.

❗ If used heavily, may rob the body of essential nutrients such as vitamins A, D, E, and K.

Zea Mays

Indian Corn

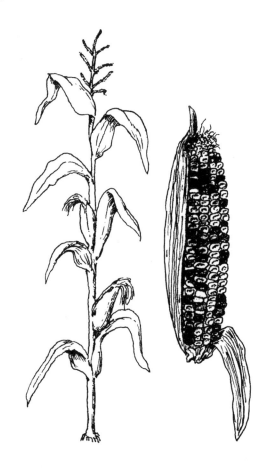

⬚ Indian corn or ornamental corn. This is the corn you can grow or purchase, that has kernels in various colors. But the herbal benefits described here apply to all corn.

☼ A summer crop that appreciates much sun and deep, rich soil for proper root development.

🌿 Use the corn silk.

🍵 While corn is certainly good for you, it is the silk that is described here for its herbal benefits. The silk is used as a diuretic that helps with urinary problems. It may be beneficial for weight loss and for controlling high blood pressure.

☞ Utilize 1 teaspoon silk to ½ cup boiling water.

❗ No cautionary concerns, except to note that, if the silk is not fresh, it may act like a very strong laxative.

JESUS AND THE HERBS

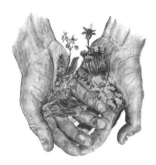

Come walk with me through a biblical herb garden.
Take a journey; note the smell, feel the textures
of the common herbs and other created things that
teach of this God who came to be with us....

I love the teachings of Jesus, especially the parables. He used common things to describe God, the kingdom of Heaven, his ministry, and our Christian walk. Certainly we can look at a rainbow and be reminded of God's promises to us. Similarly, in these pages I utilize some herbs and plants mentioned in Genesis, the Prophets, the four Gospels and in the book of Revelation to trace God's promises and warnings, Christ's ministry, and our reactions to these things.

Come along then. Place yourself back into the time that was like no time before or that will ever be again; the time when God walked among us as Jesus Christ, the Anointed One.

The Master Gardener

God said, 'Let the earth bring forth grass, the herb yielding seed, and the fruit tree yielding fruit after its kind, whose seed is in itself, upon the earth': and it was so. And the earth brought forth grass, and herb yielding seed after its kind, and the tree yielding fruit, whose seed was in itself, after its kind: and God saw that it was good. And God said, 'Behold, I have given you every herb bearing seed, which is upon the face of all the earth, and every tree, in which is the fruit of a tree yielding seed; to you it shall be for meat. And to every beast of the earth, and to every fowl of the air, and to everything that creeps upon the earth, wherein there is life, I have given every green herb for meat.'… There went up a mist from the earth, and watered the whole face of the ground. ~ Gen. 1:11-12, 29-30, 2:5-6

In Adam and Eve's day and up to Noah's day, it appears that people and animals were vegetarians. And everything in creation was good and good for you. Many scientists believe that the antediluvian earth, the one that existed before the flood of Noah, was more likely a single continent protected by a vapor canopy such as you would find in a greenhouse. The earth was watered by a system of artesian wells and high humidity. Rain and snow didn't exist. But everything flourished; plants, animals and humankind probably grew bigger, were healthier, and lived longer than they do today. Centuries-long life spans were the norm.

And the Lord God planted a garden eastward in Eden; and there he put the man whom he had formed. And out of the ground made the Lord God to grow every tree that is pleasant to the sight… And the Lord God took the man, and put him into the Garden of Eden to dress it and to keep it.
~ Gen. 2:7-9, 15 KJV

Scripture seems to indicate that the Lord God, or Jesus in his pre-incarnate state, literally planted a garden. Did he sow seeds taken from the plants he created? I suppose so. I'm sure he transplanted, separated, grafted, and maybe even weeded to place exactly what he wanted in that garden for the benefit of Adam and Eve.

As of this writing, my wife and I have moved to a new place, an acre and a half along a river. This is an untamed piece of land and I have been about the process of planting extensive gardens by clearing areas, much digging, building rock gardens, pulling some plants out, moving some, and certainly adding plants by seeding or transplanting. The work has been fun, yet arduous. I sweat and strain, yet enjoy the feel of the soil in my hands, the texture and aroma of each plant.

I think of the Lord Jesus doing something similar ages ago, and I suspect he enjoyed it much. What a God we have, willing to get down and sweat and strain with his creation!

Sometimes my two-year-old grandson comes to visit and he "helps" me in the gardens. The fruit trees we planted in the early spring—every time he comes to visit he remembers that it was he and I who planted them. I could not help but think that Adam must have looked on as the Lord God worked. How else would he have learned? Like my grandson, he watched and remembered.

Perhaps the Lord God thought, "I will place some of these grapevines here and prune them so Adam and Eve can one day have fine grapes. I will start a field of wheat here and a field of barley there, so they will never go hungry. And this would be a good place over here for an orchard of olives and over there a nice sunny spot for figs. They will appreciate that!" He planted the place in love for the creatures who bore his image.

I think of the Lord God, the pre-incarnate Jesus, walking in the garden in the cool of the day with Adam and Eve, to enjoy what he had created. They might have noted the progress of the growing plants and thought about what the garden would become and yield under his care and direction. I can imagine he and Adam talked about the plants and I am sure that there was much instruction on what to do and how to utilize what was planted.

Often, when my grandson is visiting, I gather him in my arms at the end of the day and we walk through the gardens, and I talk to him about what has been done, and how cool God is for creating all this for us. And I speak of what we have done and what will come. These are precious times for both of us. The enjoyment is written on my face and I see it on his, too. We look at the young apple trees, and he says, "Apple" and takes an imaginary bite of what will eventually come.

As you next enter your garden to work in it, may you see that picture in your mind of the Lord God tending the garden and know that you are much more precious to him than trees, shrubs, flowers, and herbs.

God finished his work in that garden, and he left it for humankind to tend. He, however, tends to *us* everyday, seeking growth, health, fruit, and a great harvest until it is time to take us home. It is not a job he finishes until we leave this earth. Can you see him weeding out of your life that which doesn't need to be there? Can you see him pruning and fertilizing and coaxing you along to be more like him and a more effective Christian for his sake?

Man's first vocation was as a gardener. One would wonder if it would be better for us all if we were to do a little gardening. Is there a value in being close to the earth, being personally involved with the produce we live by? I think so. If we are spending more time in the garden, then we are less apt to end up at the fast-food drive-through window, eating stuff that we really don't need and that has little value for us.

THE TREES IN THE GARDEN

The Lord God commanded the man, saying, 'Of every tree of the garden you may freely eat: but of the tree of the knowledge of good and evil, you shall not eat of it: for in the day you eat thereof you shall surely die.' When the woman saw that

the tree was good for food, and that it was pleasant to the eyes, and a tree to be
desired to make one wise, she took of the fruit thereof, and did eat, and gave also
unto her husband. ~ Gen. 2:16-17, 3:6 KJV

All plants were available for food, except one. What a wide variety of choices they had, and we have much of that choice today, but we limit ourselves in partaking of that abundance. Fortunately for the adventurous, there are farmer's markets, natural food grocers, and expanded produce sections in mainstream grocery stores that are offering a tremendous selection.

Why is it that we tend to mess up a good thing? God truly gave us a free lunch. But our act of disobedience and disrespect for God got us a curse. We live under that curse today, although most of the time it is pretty livable. But if you think about it, we still have the tendency to take the good things God has given us for food and make them less nutritious. Why did we decide to refine such staples as flour and rice by removing from them that which was best for us?

The generations of the 20th century have done more than any other age to turn good natural foods into stuff of little value. Maybe we can make the 21st century different, and get back closer to the plan that God had for those who lived in Eden. It doesn't make much sense to be doing all this refining that makes us sick. Then because we are sick, we add both over-the-counter and prescribed remedies to counteract the junk we eat. Combine poor and problematic foods with a lot of chemicals, and we are setting ourselves up for far more illness and misery than were necessary as a result of the "fall."

After the fall of mankind in the garden, life changed. We still had the herbs but they were a little harder to get, weren't as perfect as before, and if you weren't careful with some of them you could get stuck, stung, or very ill from eating something that now had a poisonous nature. Because of humankind's sin, corruption of all that was good became common. Life became much more difficult. Now with the good herbs came thorns and thistles, and caring for the garden became hard work. And evil was everywhere, to the point that God finally became fed up with humankind and decided to teach all but eight people to do the "dead man's float."

Again the world and the life upon it went through a cataclysmic change. Because of the flood of Noah, the world no longer housed just one continent. But more importantly, the protective vapor canopy that surrounded the earth was eliminated and the earth we now live on became the order of this present age. With the change, God changed the rules of what we could eat.

Every moving thing that lives shall be meat for you; even as the green herb
have I given you all things. ~ Gen. 9:3, KJV

We went from being herbivores to omnivores, now eating flesh too. But for God's chosen people, the Hebrews, this change came with a huge set of dietary laws meant to protect the health of the people. After the formation of the Christian church 2,000 years ago, God adjusted the rules again, placing all things that can be eaten on the "clean" list. So, God now gives you permission to eat anything that can be considered food. But that doesn't necessarily make everything good or best for you. Modern medicine is discovering that you truly are what you eat. Generally speaking, take good things in, good health results; take bad things in, bad health results.

Here is something to consider: If we are "fearfully and wonderfully made" as the Bible describes us and we are to be the living temple of the Holy Spirit and a place where Jesus comes to live happily, then shouldn't we also care about our physical well-being and be careful in what we consume?

THE HOLY SEED

So the holy seed will be the stump in the land. ~ Isa. 6:13b

Most gardeners, I suppose, look at seeds as holy in the sense that they are set apart for a great purpose. So it is something to think about Jesus as a Holy Seed. I have shared with you about his being the first gardener and the Master Gardener, but he is also the seed, the Holy Seed of God.

As long as the earth endures, seedtime and harvest, cold and heat, summer and winter, day and night will never cease. ~ Gen. 8:22

If you're like me, I know what you're thinking about during January and February: probably not the snow lying in big drifts on the ground and the short days of sunlight, but spring and seeds. More than likely your house is littered with garden catalogs full of pictures of luscious plants in full bloom and the harvest they promise. You are thinking about and ordering seeds months before the growing season begins. I'm not so sure God didn't contemplate his plan for man in the same way.

In the sixth chapter of Isaiah we see this great prophet called to duty. He is literally raptured into the throne room of God, where he sees Jehovah "high and exalted" and heavenly beings beyond our ability to imagine. And then he sees himself as we must all see ourselves eventually: "a man of unclean lips."

Isaiah also experiences God cleansing him of his sin and commissioning him to "Go and tell the people" of what is to come. At the time of Isaiah, God's creation had rolled on for four millenniums and with pretty much disastrous results because of sin. Isaiah lived after the time of Israel's glory that occured during the reigns of Kings David and Solomon. Assault after assault from the Assyrians, and then a time of captivity for the nation of Israel in evil Babylon, it looked as if God's favored people were once again nothing more than slaves and in real danger of complete destruction and extinction.

Isaiah was sent out to tell these people who were "ever hearing but not understanding" that they needed to turn from their wicked ways and be healed. And although the peoples and the lands would be decimated for a season, in a distant spring to come, a seed would be planted that would signify a new beginning. The sign of Immanuel, of a virgin birth, the promise of a seed sprouting in a barren and arid land, is given. This seed will change the world.

Seeds fascinate me. Just think how many watermelons, tomatoes, etc. one seed can provide. Maybe six to sixty. But when you think about how many more seeds each of those fruit will provide, then an infinitesimal number of watermelons and tomatoes are possible, potentially enough to stretch out through the ends of the universe and for all time. That is God's seed plan: Through his seed, Jesus Christ, scattered everywhere through and by his people, there is enough for all, for all time. In the barren desert wasteland of humanity, God shows his love to the undeserving by being willing to bless them abundantly and for eternity. He plants a seed. In fact, the Bible tells us that he *is* that seed.

In Jesus' Parable of the Sower found in Luke 8, we see a farmer out sowing seed. The seed falls in many places, such as hard paths, rocky ground, among the thorns, and also in good soil. We, of course, want to be good soil and we do this by reading and abiding in his word. God the Son is described as the word, and the Bible is also described as the word. The end of the parable tells us: "The seed is the word of God" (Lk. 8:11). God doesn't have to wait until winter to purchase, or spring to plant, his seed. He does it every time we read the Bible and abide in him, and the result is that the seed "comes up and yields a crop, a hundred times more than was sown." That is the potential for the garden of our lives, ever-bearing and always fruitful.

Jesus was very clear about his mission, even though it was hard for those at that time to understand it. We have life and can be fruitful because of the death, and yet life, of the Holy Seed.

I tell you the truth, unless a kernel of wheat falls to the ground and dies, it remains only a single seed. But if it dies, it produces many seeds. ~ Jn. 12:24

THE PROMISE

First there was a promise. For a long time it had seemed that God was absent. For centuries, no true prophet had spoken for God. It had been four hundred years since the God-breathed words of the prophet Malachi gave a hint of things to come:

But for you who revere my name, the sun of righteousness will rise with healing in its wings. And you will go out and leap like calves released from the stall. ~ Mal. 4:2

But the centuries rolled by and generations of people came and went. Maybe some folks thought God had given up on his creation. But one old man named Zechariah, a devout believer who served as a priest, waited with a glimmer of hope that God still answered prayer (read his story in Luke Chapter 1).

Hoping against hope, Zechariah desired to be a father so that he would have a son to carry on the priesthood. But the years wore on, his wife Elizabeth was barren, and time could not heal a barren womb. But much to his surprise, Elizabeth became pregnant, and Zechariah was to become a father.

Not only that. Because of his faithfulness, this aged man would sire John the Baptist, a new prophet who would finally speak for God and make the announcement for which millions had waited. For many years Zechariah had hoped and prayed for a miracle, because he knew that his only hope was a miracle from God. He didn't know, however, that God not only heard his prayer, but he would answer it in a most unique way.

And when the time for the burning of incense came, all the assembled worshipers were praying outside. ~ Lk. 1:10

It was an interesting time when Zechariah lived in Jerusalem. The city had some peace and enjoyed some prosperity; but it was a place that existed under martial law. Rome was in its dominance as the political and military power of the known world.

Pax Romana, an iron-fisted, enforced peace, ruled the day. And while the Hebrew lands were for the most part safe from their enemies, Israel was again in bondage. True, it wasn't the bondage of enslavement in foreign lands. But the Hebrew's own land was filled and ruled by foreigners. Long gone was the greatness of Kings David and Solomon.

For those who were truly looking, such as Zechariah, there was the day-to-day reminder that the promise of "God with us" had not been fulfilled. For those who sought God—and not all did—the words of Israel's greatest prophet rang in their ears:

Awake, awake, O Zion, clothe yourself with strength. Put on your garments of splendor, O Jerusalem, the holy city. The uncircumcised and defiled will not enter you again. Shake off your dust; rise up, sit enthroned, O Jerusalem. Free yourself from the chains on your neck, O captive Daughter of Zion. ~ Isa. 52:1-2

As in every land, there were groups of people who shared common bonds and beliefs. There were the Zealots—revolutionary and radical in their actions. They hoped for the warrior king who would come and kick fannies and take names and boot Rome out of the land. They waited, plotted, and sought for the "Warrior God" to appear.

Then there were the Pharisees, who believed in God—a God of rules, rites, ceremonies, and outward obedience, while inside they were nothing but "dead men's bones." But if they did just the right things in just the right order, they thought maybe the "God of Laws" would come and relieve them of the bondage.

Then there were the Sadduccees. They said they believed in God, and yet they didn't believe in an after-life. The hereafter for them was what they were "here after now." Involved in religion for what they could *get*, their God was a "Live-now God"and by using the system they could find power, position, and wealth even in times of Roman rule. They were content to live with "the God who wasn't there."

Finally, there were the Essenes (the probable writers of the Dead Sea Scrolls), a mysterious and secretive group, a splinter sect of the Pharisees. These were people who understood that God was also a God of mercy and that all the rites and rules couldn't separate them completely from their sins. They read the holy scriptures and found a God who himself would pay the cost of sin. He would be the "Sacrifice God." While they didn't understand it all, they waited for this Savior God who would somehow pay the penalty for their sins.

If we had been there, maybe we would have chosen a group to associate with. Maybe we wouldn't have known just where we stood, but somehow we also would have a nagging sense that the promise—the promise from God—was unfulfilled.

There in the sunny lands of the Hebrews, the old scriptures said that the people walked in darkness and waited for the promise. And the priests and the people prayed and the frankincense burned as if the smoke was a prayer itself that could somehow reach to God. Maybe he would hear his people.

Zechariah, serving as priest, slipped alone into the tent that was known as the Holy of Holies. In this confined space, filled with the thick smell and smoke of burning Frankincense, Zechariah's old eyes took time to adjust. Then Zechariah discovered he was not alone with the invisible presence of God.

> *Then an angel of the Lord appeared to him, standing at the right side of the altar of incense. When Zechariah saw him, he was startled and was gripped with fear. But the angel said to him: 'Do not be afraid, Zechariah; your prayer has been heard.'* ~ Lk. 1:11-13

The promise was about to be fulfilled. John would be born; and he would herald the arrival of the greatest gift of all.

THE ARRIVAL

Blessed calamity is what happened to Joseph and Mary, poor but devout people living in an out-of-the-way place called Nazareth. God would place one part of himself, as his only begotten Son, in the womb of a young teenage girl.

And it would take the strong convincing of angels to let Mary and her husband-to-be, Joseph, know that they weren't crazy or in danger of judgment, but instead highly favored of God; and that Mary's son was also to be the King-of-all-kings and the Lord-of-all-lords, the long-awaited Messiah.

But it wasn't a palace grand, draped in gold and purple cloth where this king would first lay his head. No, it would be in a wooden trough where animals came to eat. Shepherds, stunned in the fields by angels, staggered in joy to see the miracle held in a cave behind the Inn of Bethlehem. And there were a few others who came too—unlikely people as ever could a Hebrew imagine: travelers from Babylon came to worship.

Then they opened their treasures and presented him with gifts of gold and of (frank)incense and of myrrh. ~ Matt. 2:11b

You may remember, from many a Christmas pageant, this very familiar story of the Magi who came to worship and bring gifts to baby Jesus. And you are probably familiar with the gifts the Magi brought: the gold, the frankincense, and the myrrh. If you have read the sections on these herbs, then you have already learned some of the spiritual significance of them. But think of this. The creator God planned in advance the kinds of herbs that he would make available in full knowledge that they would serve a purpose for him, and that if we were looking, we could learn more of him by knowing more about the plants he created. Just as we are fearfully and wonderfully made, and God has full knowledge of our inner being (the number of our days, etc.), I believe he also created everything so that it would serve his purposes. And through these things he will be praised.

And so here are the Magi, knowing yet unknowing, star gazers from the East. Familiar enough with the scriptures of old to know that a star would herald the birth of the King. And so for a king they brought gifts. But did they understand, as we now can, the exact nature of the gifts? Did they know how these substances would tell the story of the mission and person of this newborn babe who would be King? This was the King of all kings; this was God in flesh; and this was a Lamb, the suffering sacrifice.

First, there was gold. Only kings could afford gold. So the Magi brought gold to the one who would be the King of all kings.

Secondly, the Magi brought frankincense. How the aroma must have filled the room where the Christ child lay. It was a scent that reminded everyone of God. For millenniums the prayers and the smoke had gone up to Heaven. And now God heard and answered; and God came down.

Then there was the myrrh. Its aroma mixed with the fragrance of the frankincense as the jar was opened. Myrrh was a substance used for perfume by those ladies who could afford it. But why give it to a poor babe? Its aroma would also be a reminder of the end of life, since myrrh was a key material used to treat a lifeless body—aged, worn and spent—as it was laid to rest after a lifetime was gone. Myrrh was purchased as an investment, much like our purchase of a little plot of land in the cemetery, when the realization hits us that these human suits don't last forever.

So one would think, "What a strange gift for a newborn." But it was not a strange thing to give to the one who would die for his people. Myrrh now reminds us that sin came with a price—death for the innocent and for the guilty. Even in those moments of new birth, promise and expectation, myrrh was a reminder that someone would have to die.

But at the time, baby Jesus lay in swaddling clothes, and God was with us—God in diapers. Learning to walk and talk would take time. But the promise from the long-ago days of Moses was coming true.

I will put my dwelling place among you, and I will not abhor you. I will walk among you and be your God, and you will be my people.
~ Lev. 26:11-12

The gifts had been given to him, he had received them, and now he would become the Gift. Abruptly at age thirty Jesus left the family business behind, went to the Jordan River, met his cousin John there, was baptized among the repentant, and was anointed as the Messiah. He soon found disciples for his new cause, and the ministry began. But it had a most interesting start.

THE FIRST MIRACLE

Jesus said to the servants, 'Fill the jars with water.... Now draw some out and take it to the master of the banquet.' ... Then he ... said,' you have saved the best (wine) till now.' This, the first of the miraculous signs, Jesus performed. ~ Jn. 2:7-11

While I am not a wine drinker, I certainly appreciate Jesus' first miracle. To the disciples—just beginning an incredible journey—it may have seemed a strange miracle compared with the others, which mostly had to do with healing, feeding, calming the elements, and exorcism. But upon second look, it is certainly apropos. This miracle shows the bursting excitement Christ brought when he began his ministry. His mother, Mary, may not have had all that in mind when she appealed to her son for help as the wedding feast ran out of wine; she just knew that for the moment something needed to be done, and her son could do it.

At that time, the temple worship and service to God had become mechanical and polluted. But when Jesus began his ministry, he made Jehovah real to people again. After many dry years, the idea of a Kingdom of Heaven became fresh and imminent, something to be sought and found.

So in this first miracle, water became fine wine. And it was the best a vintner could ever hope to produce, even when God, the sun and the rain had smiled upon the harvest—even when time and chance perfected a quality so pleasing to the palette that the cost went up along with the heady aroma. And so, Jesus came as the best the vine could offer; as a fine wine, the finest that could be found.

NEW WINE

And no one pours new wine into old wineskins. If he does, the new wine will burst the skins. ~ Lk. 5:37

The basics of religion had become a lot of old, dried out, parched and useless wineskins. Jesus brought new wine. The elements of a new wine will expand with power and force. The chemical reactions during the wine's fermentation will cause the substance to literally burst the materials that try to contain it.

The new mission was to bring a faith and a way to walk that you could hang your hat on. Substance is what Jesus brought. What Jesus poured upon the world was meant to burst it open. So let Jesus explode your preconceived notions about who God is, his plan and purpose, your relationship with him, and how you ought to be living.

It was new wine, it was a new day—and the old way and the new way had no way with each other ever again. Jesus came with a message that had an either/or reality to it. Be a part of it, and you will be a part of an everlasting kingdom. Don't be, and the trash heap at Gehenna might as well be your last stop.

A MAT OF REEDS

I tell you, get up, take your mat and go home. ~ Mk. 2:11

The stuff of earth can make our journey a little more comfortable. For the infirm man of Bible days, reeds and sticks meant mobility, at least with the help of a few close friends. Legs that were meant to bend—feet that were meant to walk, run, and even to dance—knew only the reeds of the mat. Yet there he was, that man mentioned in the gospel, day after day with little to do but lay upon the mat and beg for a few coins. Perhaps he thought of those reeds and remembered how God had used reeds to make a little boat to save a baby named Moses. Maybe that gave him hope that somehow God would hear his prayer and he would be given another chance.

Then came Jesus and his friends (and isn't it nice to have friends) and Jesus healed him and a new life was given, much more of a new life than the crippled man could understand at that moment. But I wonder what happened to the mat? I would have framed it and hung it on the wall for all to see. To all who would ask I would say, "Let me tell you what Jesus did for me!" What did Jesus do for *you* today? When was the last time you told someone what Jesus did for you?

THE REED

A reed swayed by the wind? ~ Matt. 11:7x

This word "reed" here is used to describe John the Baptist. His ministry may have been short, a very few years at most, like a reed that for a short season blows in the wind, briefly noticed, but soon gone. In contrast, Jesus tells us that John's faithfulness, obedience and sense of call to duty were as great as any one human had ever shown. Do you know that God has something for you to do?

Recently, as I went through the uneasy process of making a change in my ministry direction, God gave me a quiet assurance. "I have a place for you." Maybe you remember the scripture:

> But God chose the foolish things of the world to shame the wise; God chose the weak things of the world to shame the strong. ~ 1 Cor. 1:27

In the early days of my Christian walk, this verse meant much to me. If God even used foolish and weak things, then in God's plan there must be room for me.

John's short ministry may have appeared as a frail reed tossed by the wind. You, too, may feel like that reed as you consider the things God would have you do. You may ask yourself, "Can I do them?" and "Can I even live out the Christian life?" But God has a promise for you:

> ... being confident of this, that he who began a good work in you will carry it on to completion until the day of Christ Jesus. ~ Phil. 1:6

God sees what you cannot see. He sees you finishing the race set before you. His confidence, like your own confidence should be, isn't in you, but in himself carrying out the plan he has for you.

WHEAT AND CHAFF

... gathering his wheat into the barn and burning up the chaff
with unquenchable fire. ~ Matt. 3:12b

There is to be a gathering of those who choose to adopt Christ's new way. Just as there is to be a gathering of all the people who have chosen his way since the formation of the Christian faith. In the between-time of eternity to eternity, there is work to be done.

Here in the book of Matthew, you and I are described as "wheat," a useable and beneficial grain with much value. It seems most apt and most kind of Jesus, the "Bread of Life" to compliment us in such a way.

The disciples were given much to consider from the familiar things of life. How could you look at a kernel of wheat, a loaf of bread, and not think of this new way of life Jesus brought? Or for that matter, how could you think of the valueless chaff and not think of the end coming for those who would not accept the Lord's gift? At the end of harvest, the wheat is gathered in one place; then workers sift through the wheat, tossing it into the air. As the wheat is lifted high in the air with a winnowing fork and the wind catches it, the wheat will fall to the ground unaffected by the wind; but the chaff blows away from the wheat, fit only for the fire.

Wheat chaff was deemed as useless and purposeless. Chaff weighs little, whereas wheat is heavy.

Similarly, an evil man named King Belshazzar in the book of Daniel Chapter Five was found by God to be useless and wanting. God's finger reached from Heaven, and on a wall wrote these words, "Mene, Mene, Tekel, Parsinin."

The great and humble prophet Daniel was the only one who could interpret the words; but the interpretation would bring Belshazzar to his knees and to ruin as well. The most powerful king in the world at that time was at the end of his days. He may have thought it was party time; but his kingdom was at an end, and when the value of the life he had lived was weighed in the scales, it was like chaff—useless to God and of no purpose.

It must have meant great things to the disciples to hear that they were to be like wheat, full of goodness and purpose, ready to be reaped and brought to God's storehouse.

We face a decision. We can come to the warehouse, be filled with the goodness of Christ—or remain as chaff. Like chaff, at the end of this short life, we have nothing to look forward to but the fire—we have judged ourselves; we are gone from God's sight. But unlike the chaff, we face an eternal torment for our decision.

FASTING AND OIL

But when you fast, put oil on your head and wash your face ...
~ Matt. 6:17

Christ's new wine called for sacrifice—his upon the cross, and ours in carrying our cross daily. As you seek God's purpose in your life, the move to holiness takes time. There is so much stuff of ourselves to come to terms with and to clear away. Fasting, the act of cutting off from yourself the things you are accustomed to every day, can help in the cleansing process.

The age-old tradition of fasting, though, had lost its meaning and purpose at the time Jesus stepped into our world.

God questions us in so many words: "Are you going to fast? Then do it for the right purpose, to draw closer to me, not to show others how self-righteous you are. You are not some sort of holy honcho just because for a few hours you decide to go without. If you seek me through fasting, be of good cheer about it; because suffering for Christ isn't really suffering at all, and it will draw you closer to me."

Walking on the way with Christ means giving up in order to receive. Letting go of everything helps you realize just how much you really have. Without all the clutter around you to block your view, then you can really see all the things God has provided for you.

GRASS AND LILIES

See how the lilies of the field grow ... [and] the grass of the field. ~ Matt. 6:28, 30x

I love the wildflowers in spring and summer. I go out to the Lava Beds National Monument in the high desert country of northeastern California to see the wildflowers. And I like to watch the grasses in summer and fall sway with the winds on the bluffs above the sea on the Oregon Coast.

Out in the harsh desert land of the lava beds and the windy places at land's edge, spectacular arrays and varieties of wildflowers bloom in all colors, hues, shapes, and sizes, including wild lilies. My favorite happens to be a wildflower called Indian paintbrush, which often grows in abundance. Dashed in oranges and yellows, this distinctive plant reminds me of the intricacy of God's character and creative power. In this seemingly-stark land, God has provided just the right climate and conditions for a great, natural rock garden.

The message was the same for those who followed Jesus. To them he says:

Look around, can anything be more beautifully adorned and cared for than the lilies of the field? Even the raiment of the richest king in the world, King Solomon, couldn't even compare! ~ Matt. 6:28-29, author's paraphrase

This is the message to the disciples and to us:

But seek first his kingdom and his righteousness, and all these things will be given to you as well. ~ Matt. 6:33

God has promised us an abundance; our needs (not our wants) will be taken care of. To become a disciple, or follower, of Christ meant to step out of where you were to follow a new path. John, James, and Peter left their fishing nets. Matthew left the lucrative, knife-to-your-back business of taxation without representation. These men needed to see it differently. "Look," God is saying, "lift your eyes, see the lilies and the grasses along the way; and if I will clothe them in this beauty, then will I not clothe you, feed you, care for you on your way to my righteousness!"

GOOD FRUIT

Do people pick grapes from thornbushes, or figs from thistles? ... A good tree cannot bear bad fruit. ~ Matt. 7:16, 18a

If you look in Genesis and read about creation, you will notice this recurring theme: the things God created—from seeds and plants to animals—were created "according to their kind." Apple trees were created to produce apples, deer were created to produce more deer. Adam named them all. A cow was a cow, a plesiosaur was a plesiosaur and a sparrow a sparrow, and that would be all they ever would be.

But these words also come as a warning for us to watch out for wolves in sheep's clothing. The fruit one bears tells of the nature of the person.

Jesus bore much good fruit. Whether you choose to believe that he is God and Savior, you can't fault him; he bore only good fruit through his character, work, and mission.

The question we are left with then is twofold: First, with whom do we associate, and do they bear good fruit? Second, if we associate with Christ and call him our own, do we now bear good fruit?

Looking at the early days of the disciples, one may not see good fruit in them. John and James, the Sons of Thunder, vied for the best place next to Jesus. Peter, loud and emotional, wanted to start an uprising in Gethsemene, but later shrank back in cowardice at the sound of a rooster heralding a dark day. And then there was Doubting Thomas. Faith and doubt—how can that work?

But with the Holy Spirit at Pentecost, these disciples were changed for all time. Their new lives bore good fruit and we are the result of their mission. The fruit they bore is described as "... love, joy, peace, patience, kindness, goodness, faithfulness, gentleness and self-control" (Gal. 5:22-23a). Through the power of the Holy Spirit, utilizing our gifts, we are to bear much fruit also. So if we are to bear much fruit, then why do we read what we see next!

THE HARVEST

The harvest is plentiful but the workers are few. ~ Matt. 9:37

Have you ever been caught up in a multi-level marketing business? Some are good, many are bad, but these businesses and their successes are based not only on product quality and marketability, but on your enthusiasm for the product. The product may be great; but the prosperity you seek only comes to you based upon what you do with the business. How much of the product will you use? How well will you convince others to use it?

Then isn't it fascinating that God brings to us a life of incredible proportions that we can enjoy today and for all eternity; nothing really compares with it; and yet the harvest dies in the field! He asks us to participate in showing this life to others. And why would we not want to? Yet from the days of Jesus' ministry, in the early churches of Acts, and through the centuries to now, those who need to know—those who need to be gathered like the wheat and brought into the Lord's storehouse—remain in the field because there aren't enough workers. Or maybe the problem is there aren't enough motivated workers willing to see the need of bringing in the harvest before it is forever lost.

I wonder. Do we think maybe there isn't enough of God to go around, so we hoard his grace, too selfish to share? Maybe it is fear that keeps us down? Maybe we don't think we know all we should and are waiting to finish up one more Bible study or to be encouraged by another sermon?

Paul found an exception that seems to supersede any excuse we can come up with. He gives a great description of those who are the workers and what motivates them. This great missionary and church planter set up churches everywhere he could. He worked hard and did great things. But he faced what many of us in ministry have faced at times—little appreciation and reciprocation for his efforts. However, he found one group, the Philippians, to be different. They were concerned for Paul and for his ministry and the others he sought to help. He says of the Christians in Philippi: "Indeed, you have been concerned.... You sent me aid again and again when I was in need" (Phil. 4:10, 16).

Maybe the reason the fields are ready for harvest and yet lack workers to harvest them comes down to that one word, *concern*.

Do we care enough, do we show the fruit of the Christian life? Are we truly concerned about the hurting and lost? Do we look at them and realize that if we do not show them the Christ that they may be lost forever or do we think somebody else will do it?

I can remember my conversion process. It came later in life. I was basically hell's statistic and the devil's gain. There is a tractable time; then when you pass a certain age the likelihood of Christian conversion becomes more remote as the years go by. I had passed a certain age when most people are saved. And if it hadn't been for a few faithful people who wouldn't give up on me, but kept witnessing to me, praying for me, and admonishing me, I believe I would have been lost. They made the difference. I became saved and another kernel of wheat was brought in; and my life did not become like chaff.

Why did they do it for me? Bottom line: They were concerned.

GRAIN

His disciples were hungry and began to pick some heads of grain and eat them. ~ Matt. 12:1x

Do rules surpass need, or does need surpass rules?

Jesus came to set the captives free, to de-regulate *religion* and instigate *relation*. Jesus and the disciples were busy, there were souls to save and much work to be done and they were often so busy that they had little time for themselves and their own personal needs. So on a busy Sabbath, when the disciples came across a field of grain, and as they moved through it, they ate of its abundance. The Pharisees, like dogs on their heels, were quick to criticize. "These men are working on the Sabbath!" they screamed.

But Christ came to set us free to have joy on the journey. Our relationship with God sets us free, free indeed, and it is to be a relationship enjoyed. God is with us! Can anything be more wonderful than that? Let's not complicate this life by unnecessary rules that move us away from true worship rather than closer to worship.

ANOTHER REED

A bruised reed he will not break. ~ Matt. 12:20 (quoting Isaiah)

Not only did Jesus compare John the Baptist to a swaying reed, but he also told how he would treat a bruised reed. This fragile plant that can be broken by the wind would not be injured by the all-powerful God. The prophet Isaiah tells that Jesus came in mercy and grace—not to harm, but to heal and to preserve.

What does Jesus see when he sees us? Sometimes I fear that he sees a sinner that just needs a good toasting, and judgment waits for me regardless of my efforts to be like him. But I must not let condemnation get in the way of love. Love is God's motivation. Nothing but love would endure so much.

I love the county fairs in summer, especially the animal exhibits. I like to see the 4-H kids tending their animals of choice. Young girls with little lambs, caring for them as if they were small children or toy baby dolls. Lambs are a good example of the fact that something can be as dumb as a stick and yet cute. The word tells us God sees us as "harassed and helpless, like sheep without a shepherd" (Matt. 9:36). Without Jesus, there is no chance for us in this world. He is the one who will keep us from the predators the devil sends out to devour the sheep.

The ultimate act of Jesus' love for us comes in the form of the cross. Without doubt, nothing compares to that act of love. But there is another act that never leaves my mind. That is his act of not only not harming a bruised reed, but his loving act of cleansing it and healing it.

> *A man with leprosy came and knelt before him and said, 'Lord, if you are willing, you can make me clean.' Jesus reached out his hand and touched the man. 'I am willing,' he said. 'Be clean!'* ~ Matt. 8:2-3

Here was a man deformed beyond recognition by a horrible disease. An outcast, unloved but by those who suffered with him. All the promise life held was lost when a couple of whitish, scaley blotches appeared on his skin. Death had won again—only the dying went on for years, and it came with loneliness and expulsion from society.

If this man was outside of the leper colonies, traveling, and other "clean" people approached, he would have to shout at the top of his lungs, "Unclean, unclean." This way, people would be warned to stay away. In Jewish law, it was forbidden to touch a leper. This man, that no one would have touched with a ten-foot pole, reached out to Jesus. And Jesus reached out to him, made effort and touched and cured him. That is love.

The Seeds

> *A farmer went out to sow his seed.... Some seed fell among thorns. But the worries of this life and the deceitfulness of wealth choked it, making it unfruitful.* ~ Matt. 13:3, 7, 22
> *The farmer sows the word.* ~ Mk. 4:13-14

One of my greatest joys is seeing a new seed sprout when a person becomes a new Christian. It is always amazing. Something clicks in the life of this person, and he or she becomes God-aware. It is like a flower coming to bloom. His or her life becomes Christ-rich in color, hue and texture.

But one of my greatest sorrows is to see this person lose that first love; the things of the world encroach back on him. Before you know it, she has reverted to her old self. For some reason, he decides that God isn't enough. I have seen some drastic changes in people who go to God—and then amazingly enough, back from God. I am always astounded. "What in this life compares with the glories of God in our lives?" I ask myself. And yet some turn away, resort to the cheap thrills of this world, and I am left shaking my head, thinking, "You have given God up for *this*?"

THE TARES

His enemy came and sowed weeds among the wheat. ~ Matt. 13:26

The other word for weeds here is "tares." Tares look like wheat when first planted. They masquerade as the real thing. But if you are fooled into thinking they are the real thing and consume them, you will be poisoned. It is this way with the false churches. You have probably had friendly people show up at your doorstep to share Christ with you. Or "spiritually-enlightened" friends share their beliefs with you. But often this is a very different God with a very different "gospel." We must always be on guard for the tares, because they can and will in astonishing numbers succeed in drawing people away from the true God, poisoning with the false one.

MUSTARD

The kingdom of heaven is like a mustard seed.... Though it is the smallest of all your seeds, yet when it grows, it is the largest of garden plants and becomes a tree, so that the birds of the air come and perch in its branches.
~ Matt. 13:31-32

No other Bible verse meant more to me as a child than this one. I remember receiving a card from my Sunday school teacher upon my childhood conversion (which, by the way, I walked away from for twenty years). In the card was a little mustard seed, barely visible, taped into the card. This little seed was given in faith by a caring Sunday school teacher who prayed for me, and the Lord kept his hand on me.

I like to grow mustard in the garden. But I always grow too much. The little seeds are incredible in the amount and size of plants they produce. God gives us a seed of faith, a deposit. Nourished by the Bread of Life and the Living Water, this seed can grow abundantly. Sunday school teachers are wonderful in that way. They plant a lot of seed and the results can be phenomenal.

I tell you the truth, if you have faith as small as a mustard seed, you can say to this mountain, 'Move from here to there,' and it will move. ~ Matt. 17:20

Miracles still happen; and when Jesus said that we can move mountains, I believe he literally meant it. Sometimes I think the march of ministry through the centuries is slow. But then I think of groups of people like the Pilgrims, the first missionaries in Africa and China, the early days of The Salvation Army ... and there is no doubt that the Lord has allowed the faithful to move mountains, when they have believed that they can.

YEAST

Be on your guard against the yeast of the Pharisees and Sadducees.
~ Matt. 16:6

Have you ever put too much yeast in a recipe and had it literally blow up what you were baking? Or have you put in too little yeast or yeast that was old, and didn't get any of the rising effects? Yeast is meant to invade a substance. But in this context Jesus sees the yeast as a negative (note Matt. 16:12). He was not telling his listeners to guard against the yeast used in bread, but against the teaching of the Pharisees and Sadducees which Jesus saw as a foreign substance that would ruin the true essence of the Word and the purposes of God.

Consider the yeast of the hypocrites and its damaging effect upon the bread. Then, let's compare that with what the Creator can do with a helpful little boy's gift of a few loaves of barley bread.

BARLEY

When I broke the five loaves for the five thousand, how many basketfuls of pieces did you pick up? ~ Mk. 8:19
So they gathered them and filled twelve baskets with the pieces of the five barley loaves left over. ~ Jn. 6:13

How could such a thing happen? Jesus took a few loaves of bread and began to break it into pieces; but instead of getting a dozen or so pieces, enough for one person, he kept breaking until five thousand men plus their wives and children and other relatives had enough to eat, along with the disciples. Enough was left over to fill twelve baskets.

If you try to understand how such a phenomenon could have happened, then you miss the value of the miracle. It happened because he who made the universe by thinking it into existence can do those things that are impossible for us to do or even to consider doing. You may have heard it said, "Bread is the staff of life." We can fuel our bodies and keep them alive for a while. But we must seek the eternal life, too—and so we need Jesus. For the bread of God is he who comes down from Heaven and gives life to the world.

Then Jesus declared, 'I am the bread of life. He who comes to me will never go hungry, and he who believes in me will never be thirsty.'
~ Jn. 6:35

Fig

Seeing a fig tree by the side of the road, he went up to it but found nothing on it except leaves. Then he said to it, 'May you never bear fruit again!' Immediately the tree withered. ~ Matt. 21:18-19
Yet I hold this against you: You have forsaken your first love. Remember the height from which you have fallen! Repent and do the things you did at first. ~ Rev. 2:4-5

This is a curious miracle because it shows Jesus in what appears to be a harsh light. Utilizing a parable as a teaching tool, he places a curse on a fig tree that has leafed out but has not produced fruit. Fig trees produce their fruit before the leaves come out, so by the time a fig tree has got its leaves for the season, the fruit should be in place. Jesus knew by looking at this particular tree, that it was barren.

Maybe you have had that happen. You grow a fruit tree, it grows fine and tall with beautiful foliage, but produces no fruit. And you eventually dig it out.

Jesus had just come from the temple. He was angry that the house of God had been turned into a marketplace run by a den of thieves. They were not producing fruit. The fig tree represents this barrenness. If something won't produce, then get rid of it. It's a harsh lesson. But in the kingdom of God, productivity counts.

The Pharisees and the Sadducees were not producing, and soon their rule would wither away and end. In the book of Revelation, Jesus describes the church of Ephesus. He speaks of the great things they have done in the past;

but something has happened and they have moved away from what is really important. They are no longer producing the kind of fruit that is expected and needed.

How do we remain faithful? By remembering our first love, Jesus Christ, and ordering our steps after his.

THE SAMARITAN'S OIL AND WINE

He went to him and bandaged his wounds, pouring on oil and wine.
~ Lk. 10:34

Here we see the substances of grape and olive oil used in the healing of one who is wounded. You probably remember the story. Jesus is asked, "Who is my neighbor?" In answer, he tells the story of a man traveling from Jerusalem to Jericho, who is attacked, robbed, and severely beaten by robbers. Two priests pass by the man but do not assist him. Finally a third traveler, a Samaritan, stops to help the man. Samaritans were looked down on by the Hebrews, and vice versa. Both ethnic groups were openly hostile to each other. It was nothing more than early racism.

But this "Good Samaritan" was moved to compassion. He ministered to the man, transported him to an inn, and paid for his room and care. There was no question in this man's mind that all people should be considered our neighbors. That was the point of Jesus' lesson. We are all neighbors. We are in fact our brothers' keepers. If we don't care for them, who will?

May we be reminded that—just as the Samaritan poured the olive oil and grape wine on the injured man to treat him—so we need to pour on kindness to the Who-so-evers, regardless of who they are. I don't know if you have ever thought about it this way; but if we all came from one set of parents, Adam and Eve (and science is well on its way to proving this), then are we not all brothers and sisters?

THE VINEYARD

There was a landowner who planted a vineyard. He put a wall around it, dug a winepress in it, and built a watchtower. Then he rented the vineyard to some farmers and went away on a journey. ~ Matt. 21:33

In this story we see a picture of God, who has given the care of a well-prepared and prized vineyard to the people. They are there to take care of it and be good stewards. Instead, these ingrates take it for themselves. They will not share the harvest. They beat and kill the servants sent by God to collect some of the produce. Finally, the son of the landowner, who we now understand to be Jesus, is sent. But they kill him too.

Therefore I tell you that the kingdom of God will be taken away from you and given to a people who will produce its fruit. ~ Matt. 21:43

This story illustrates not only the fall from grace of the religious leaders of Jesus' earthly days, but also the promise of the formation of a new church—the Christian movement that has now proceeded for twenty centuries. The church must be faithful to remember that it is Christ we serve. We are not to take for granted, or take for ourselves, that over which God has assigned us to be stewards and caretakers.

The Tithe of Mint, Dill and Cumin

You give a tenth of your spices—mint, dill and cummin. But you have neglected the more important matters of the law—justice, mercy and faithfulness. ~ Matt. 23:23

Did you hear the story of the twenty dollar bill and the one dollar bill? The two bills were catching up on old times. The one dollar bill asked, "What have you been up to?"

"Oh, I've been having a great time—restaurants, movies, night clubs and cruises," replied the twenty. He then asked, "How about you?"

The one dollar bill answered, "Oh, the same old thing: church, church, church."

Christ gave his all. Do we think a little loose change, placed in an offering plate is all that is asked of us? How much is too much to give for the ministries of the Lord? I don't think there is a set amount, but we are to be imitators of Christ.

"But I don't have much money," you say. What about the intangibles that we can give? Did not God give you time, talents, treasures, and gifts which you have the ability to share?

Figs and Oil Speak of Last Things

As Jesus was sitting on the Mount of Olives, the disciples came to him privately. 'Tell us, when will this happen, and what will be the sign of

your coming and of the end of the age?'
'Now learn this lesson from the fig tree: As soon as its twigs get tender and
leaves come out, you know that summer is near.' ~ Matt. 24:3, 32

We are on a crash course with destiny, God's destiny. However, are we mistakenly thinking of time in terms of eons and billions of years? Do we think that life just goes on and on the way it is? Or do we realize that we have each been placed on a timeline? We live in the age of grace now, and it is but one of the ages that God has ordained. There was the age of Adam and Eve; then the age of the patriarchs and the age of the law. But there are other ages to come.

The Bible speaks of a seven-year tribulation that will shake many people out of their preconceived notions about time and space. It speaks of an age of the millennium, a thousand-year reign of Christ on earth. And finally, it tells us of an endless age that goes on forever for those who live today for Jesus. We need to see time as God sees it.

The foolish ones said to the wise, 'Give us some of your oil; our lamps are
going out.' ~ Matt. 25:8

Clay, olive oil, and bits of reed were the substances used for keeping a house lit after dark. It's hard for us to imagine in these days of bright lights everywhere. But when you depend upon such simple substances to chase off the darkness, you never want to find yourself without a lamp, reed, and oil—just like you don't want to miss paying the electricity bill today.

In this story, the foolish and lazy virgins miss the bridegroom because they are not prepared for his arrival. They miss out—and are locked out—forever. Time is of the essence. We, also, must wait for the Bridegroom's arrival, every day expecting Jesus to come. Perhaps it will be today. If we are left outside without oil in our lamps, then we will become lost.

Your word is a lamp to my feet and a light for my path. ~ Ps. 119:105

Like being lost on a mountain trail at night with no flashlight, without the light of the Word and the oil of the Holy Spirit we quickly lose our way in life's journey. When Jesus returns from out of the sky to place his feet once again in the Garden of Gethsemane, it will be the end of one age. A new age will have come. Be ready!

NARD

Then Mary took about a pint of pure [spike]nard, an expensive perfume;

she poured it on Jesus' feet and wiped his feet with her hair. And the house
was filled with the fragrance of the perfume. ~ Jn. 12:3

There are a couple of instances mentioned in the Bible where a woman named Mary or an unidentified woman anointed Jesus. It is believed that the incidents were performed by Mary Magdalene and/or Mary of Bethany; although it could have been another who performed this act of love and understanding.

This woman took the best she had to offer. She used it all, then she used her hair to wipe Jesus' feet. Mary would have paid dearly for this material, and normally it would have been kept in an alabaster box. The nard was used for special occasions only. Certainly having the Lord in her house was the most special occasion she had ever experienced.

Mary Magdalene is thought to have been a former prostitute. If this is true, she was a woman who knew sin as a lifestyle and profession, but the Lord got her attention. She was moved by his power and by his grace. This act of worship was an acceptance on her part that "This is my Lord." Life would change now, and whatever she owned was now for the Lord's use. Spikenard would normally have been used sparingly, but she used it all. Jesus saw this as a prophetic act that spoke of his death and atonement. We don't know whether Mary understood enough of Jesus' mission to realize that he planned to die for the world and for her; but certainly her incredible act of selfless love, stirred by having the Christ in her presence, directed her to anoint him in such a way.

You did not put oil on my head, but she has poured perfume on my feet.
Therefore, I tell you, her many sins have been forgiven—for she loved much.
~ Lk. 7:46-47

Jesus' response to Mary is what we love about this God we serve. He loved her first, even though she was a sinner living outside of God's law. And so she responded with love, and she became forgiven of her sins. It was mutual love that saved her. God loved first, regardless of her sins. She chose to express love back with the anointing nard, and also by becoming obedient. True love obeys. It is one thing to say, "I love you." But it is a very different thing to prove it. The spikenard is a reminder that it costs to follow Jesus. It may not cost money or things, but always it will cost the willingness to give obedience.

PALM

A very large crowd spread their cloaks on the road, while others cut [palm]
branches from the trees and spread them on the road. ~ Matt. 21:8

For three years Jesus had ministered in word and deed. There was no one greater than he. Even the elements listened to him and obeyed; and even the dead responded and lived again. Those who had been there when Lazarus was raised could not doubt that "Truly God" stood among them, because after a person had been dead three days and rotting in a cave, death was irreversible. But that is the point about God—He can reverse what is irreversible. He gave Mary and Martha their brother back.

Then Jesus went on to Jerusalem, the City of Peace where there was no peace, the City of the King that had no true king. But as Jesus and his disciples, accompanied by a large crowd, made their way to the city for Passover, something happened. An election was held on the streets and the ballot boxes were ripped from the date palm trees and with palm branches waving, the people ordained Jesus as the king.

The red carpet was not out; but the long, full and stately palm branch would serve well in the excitement of the procession. This was a man who could feed the multitudes, calm the seas, and even raise the dead!

It is no coincidence that more ornamental palms are sold at Easter than any other time of the year. Do we buy them just because they are nice; or is it our own way of expressing who is our eternal and personal King?

Drink This and Remember

I will not drink of this fruit of the vine from now on until that day when I drink it anew with you in my Father's kingdom. ~ Matt. 26:28

I love church potlucks—good food, great selection, and wonderful fellowship—especially at country churches. I wonder what it might have been like to have been a disciple and share an evening meal with Jesus after a long, busy day. It would finally be time to get off your feet and enjoy an intimate meal with the Lord away from the crush of the crowds. With time to enjoy it, the food would taste even better and the words of the Master, in those restful moments, would be even more satisfying.

But on the Passover night, the last night before the cross, Jesus said to his disciples, "I have eagerly awaited to eat this Passover with you." As a disciple, you would know that somehow this night was different. The rush of events told you so; but here were quiet moments, moments which Jesus looked forward to as much as you did.

How wonderful to be there in the upper room with him, in comfortable surroundings, with other men who had become friends, eating traditional foods that spoke of history and the providence of God. The best of the vine would be offered, maybe something you couldn't enjoy again for another year. And yet on this night when many startling words would be heard and events would take place, Jesus said something that would strike fear into your heart. He said he would not drink of this vine until you were gathered together in Heaven! He would not drink, thus you would not drink, and death stood in the doorway between earth and Heaven.

THORNS

They stripped him and put a scarlet robe on him, and then twisted together a crown of thorns and set it on his head. They put a staff in his right hand and knelt in front of him and mocked him. ~ Matt. 27:29

We are told that creation itself moans because of the curse put upon us. Everything bears the mark of humankind's sin. I don't know how to understand it—but I believe plants, animals, and all of creation respond in some way to the God who made them. If a thorn bush could think, I wonder how it might have mourned to know that its branches were used to hurt the very One who had made it. If a bush could have shed tears rather than causing blood to be shed, and a bush could choose, I wonder whether the bush would have chosen tears.

MYRRH AND HYSSOP

They offered him wine mixed with myrrh, but he did not take it. ~ Mk. 15:23
They ... put the sponge on a stalk of the hyssop plant, and lifted it to Jesus' lips. ~ Jn. 19:29

Jesus hung upon the cross. Death was but minutes away. The victim's tongue was swollen and pushing between his lips and an insatiable thirst prevailed. It was the pain of the execution at its worst. Every breath labored; bones, joints, nerves, tendons and muscles screamed in agony. Even the hardened, cruel Roman executioners could barely handle the sight.

As a common practice in those last minutes, strong wine and myrrh were offered as a sedative. In this way, in the final fleeting moments of life, dying wouldn't hurt so much. But Jesus refused it flat out. Why? Isaiah tells us that Jesus was the guilt offering, to be cut off from the land of the living. He was to be smitten, pierced and crushed for our iniquities, so that we could have peace. This was a moment of love, and Christ would feel all the pain for us and suffer because he loved us and he would do it without benefit of the narcotic effects of the herbs.

SPICES

When the Sabbath was over, Mary Magdalene, Mary the mother of James, and Salome bought spices so that they might go to anoint Jesus' body. ~ Mk. 16:1

Because the Sabbath lasted from Friday evening until Saturday evening, there was little time for proper anointing of Jesus' body for permanent burial. The women who loved Jesus came at first light on Sunday morning to finish the task. They brought aloes, myrrh, and other substances to anoint and to preserve the body. Though there was no embalming, the preparation was done out of respect and custom. For the women it may have been an opportunity for one last glimpse of the one who had been so full of life and seemed to have life itself in the palm of his hands. They hoped that the guards would roll away the heavy stone and allow them into the cool, dark cave.

It seemed as if the women were the first ones up and wanting to attend to the body of Jesus. Certainly it was a great act of love. They planned to wash the body and treat the skin with the spices, finally wrapping the limp form in linen with pounds of spices rolled in. But of course this did not happen. In fact if it had happened—if the women had treated the dead body of Jesus—then he would not have been God at all, just another god that wasn't.

Have you ever thought how different the world would be if this man Jesus had died and not resurrected to life? First of all, you would not be reading this book, and I would not have anything to write about. Why write about some obscure religious movement that lasted but a few years? The event probably wouldn't even have been remembered in history.

Whether you choose to believe that you are—or are not—affected by Christianity, the reality is that your way of life, where you live, the calendar that marks your days, the laws, hospitals, social movements, etc. that influence and affect your life exist because the grave could not hold Jesus.

Even though the tides turned against Jesus after the gala celebration and exuberance of Palm Sunday—even though the cross may have claimed the King for a moment—it was only for a moment. I have always thought how wonderful it must have been on that first Palm Sunday to see Jesus and to know that in my heart I would have wanted him to be the King of all kings, to be the Lord of all lords, and to pledge my allegiance from that day forth.

But because the event took place, I still can make that affirmation today. He can still be the King of my life, the Lord of my way, the God who is with me. And when I accept him in that way, acknowledge my failures and my need of a King of mercy and power, then there will be a day when I can celebrate as they did on the first Palm Sunday. In fact, a resurrection is coming for me. His new life is my new life, and he is the first fruits of that great promise of future life everlasting.

172

The Final Harvest

There before me was a great multitude that no one could count, from every nation, tribe, people and language, standing before the throne and in front of the Lamb. They were wearing white robes and were holding palm branches in their hands. And they cried out in a loud voice: 'Salvation belongs to our God, who sits on the throne, and to the Lamb.' ~ Rev. 7:9-10

Can we look at this loving experiment of creation as a growing season? Out of eternity God did something that he didn't need to do but desired to do: create us. These days, most of us who plant gardens do so not because we need to, but because we want to. For me, other than the ongoing discovery and interest of the herbs that God created for our benefit, gardening is dirt therapy and a way to unwind and debrief after a work day. This gardening process has a daily purpose and goal. Daily it gives me pleasure and exercise. And along the way I reap early benefits of radishes, spinach and lettuce. They are early performers, but I wait for a greater harvest. All my work in the spring and summer months is geared to the harvest of fall; hoping and working for fat red tomatoes, more zucchini than I can ever hope to use; baskets of apples, peaches, grapes, and plums; jars and freezer bags full of peas, corn, beans, pickled beets, and cucumbers; enough, I hope, to last me through the winter.

And then winter does come, the long dark days, rains, snows, and much time for me to look out the window and wish I could speed the winter season along. Time to plan for another season of sowing and planting, nurturing and weeding, and then finally realizing another harvest.

As the Master Gardener, does God look at the scene described above in Revelation 7:9&10 as the great harvest? All that he has created and planted, pruned and nurtured, watered and fed, trained and instructed has now been harvested, a great multitude. It is a harvest with many voices but yet one voice. It is a harvest that has accepted the love and discipline of the Creator, Caretaker and Gardener. It has chosen not to be a wild branch, but one that was willing to be conformed in and by the Master's hand.

So we must carry on enjoying the love of the Lord and enduring his discipline, knowing that we need it and that it is for a greater good, the end result being that we are counted in the multitude of that last and great harvest.

No discipline (or pruning) *seems pleasant at the time, but painful. Later on, however, it produces a harvest of righteousness and peace for those who have been trained by it. ~ Heb. 12:11*

While I might have loved to have been there on that first Palm Sunday, I do plan to be there on the great day when the Lamb takes his rightful throne. Somewhere in the crowds, in a huge multitude, I'll wave a palm branch, with tears in my eyes, joy and praise in my voice, and I'll truly see the salvation I have lived in faith for. There will be nothing greater, no moment in my time that will compare to this moment. I hope you will be there too. Will you be one of the multitude that cries out undying devotion to the Lamb: "Salvation belongs to you, you who sit upon the throne, you who are my God and my Lamb forever and ever!"

THE INVITATION

For as the soil makes the sprout to come up and a garden causes the seeds to grow, so the Sovereign Lord will make righteousness and praise spring up before all nations. ~ Isa. 61:11

Do you know Jesus? Do you know him personally, one to one, like you know your spouse, your children, friends and co-workers? Think of Adam and Eve in the garden, in the cool of the day, walking with the Lord. They saw God daily, talked with him and spent time with him in the same way that they knew each other. We know him now as Jesus Christ, the founder of the Christian church, the Savior of humankind. And he wants to have a relationship with you, up close and personal.

Most likely you have heard the expression, "born again." This is the relationship that I am talking about, a born-again relationship with God the Creator. He is a personal God who comes to live with you in your heart, closer than a friend. In this relationship you are made new and given that spiritual aspect of you that has been missing. You become a new person.

When Adam and Eve sinned by disobeying God it set a course of destruction for humankind, a death sentence. And every human being born after has been missing an important element. We are born physical, intellectual, and emotional beings. We think and feel, and we may think that that is what life is all about. But the part of us that is missing is the spiritual aspect. One great writer described it as a God-shaped emptiness in our heart that only God can fill.

Along with this condition, we also do things we know are wrong and we are guilty of these. This willful nature of ours separates us from God who is a holy God and does no wrong. This imperfection in us, this condition separates us from God. But this is not what he wants, he seeks a relationship where he is our God and we are his people. We can only have this when we choose to let God have our life. We do this through a commitment to Jesus Christ. We do this because he is the one who came and lived with us and then died for us, doing something for us that we cannot do on our own. If sin separates, and we are all sinners, and sin is a death sentence, then we are faced with a hopeless condition. We live a short life, we do things we know we shouldn't do but seem powerless to stop it, and then we die and are separated from God forever.

Jesus, however, comes to offer life and one that lasts forever and ever. This life is available to us by recognizing, admitting, and then committing. First of all we recognize that there is a God and none of us are him. We recognize that our lives, while busy, are truly empty without him. We admit our need for God, we admit that we need a Savior to die for us if we ever hope to do something about the sin nature that holds us back. When we have come to that realization, we then commit our lives to God just like a garden might commit itself to the tending of the gardener. When we commit ourselves to Jesus Christ, he takes on that responsibility with both the present and eternity in mind. I like what the first Psalm says:

> *Blessed is the man who does not walk in the counsel of the wicked or stand in the way of sinners or sit in the seat of mockers. But his delight is in the law of the Lord, and on his law he meditates day and night. He is like a tree planted by steams of water, which yields it fruit in season and whose leaf does not wither. Whatever he does prospers. ~ Ps. 1:1-3*

God does not make it hard for us to find him. We simply:

1. Admit that we are sinners.
2. Repent or turn away from our sins.
3. Recognize our need for God and acknowledge his love for us upon the cross.
4. Pray and ask him to come into our heart.
5. Seek to serve him through prayer, study of his Word and involvement in a Bible-believing church.
6. Look forward to having Jesus live within us and prepare us for a grand eternity with him!

THE TREE OF LIFE

> *To him who overcomes, I will give the right to eat from the tree of life, which is in the paradise of God ... down the middle of the great street of the city. On each side of the river stood the tree of life, bearing twelve crops of fruit, yielding its fruit every month. And the leaves of the tree are for the healing of the nations. ~ Rev. 2:7, 22:2*

Let me ask you this: What do you think happens when you get to Heaven? The Bible tells us much about our eternity of living with God and it seems that the new world being prepared for us will be like Eden revisited, but much, much better. And in this New Jerusalem (the City of Peace) we will enjoy food!

This Tree of Life is not just symbolic in that the faithful will have eternal life with Christ, but it is an actual species of tree with fruit that we will be able to consume. This glimpse of Heaven seems to indicate that we will consume fruit, it will mean good health for us, and the leaves will have a healing nature. Creation will have come full circle from the time when God created all the herbs for healing and health and pronounced that creation good. And it is great to see that even in the heavenly splendor, this great paradise, the herbs will do the same there for us as they can do now: promote health and healing.

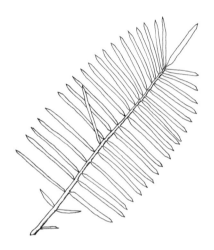

Herb Growers and Enthusiasts Across the Country

Tips and Recipes

There are many herb growers and manufacturers across the country, most of them reputable, some of them not. In order to help you explore the world of herbs a little more effectively, the next pages are contributed by participating and trustworthy herb growers and enthusiasts across the country. Many of these people share in similar beliefs that the God of the Bible created the herbs for our physical, emotional, and spiritual benefit. I included the following because of their willingness to share recipes that you may find useful and enjoyable. Here you will find information about their businesses plus some of their favorite herbs, uses, and recipes.

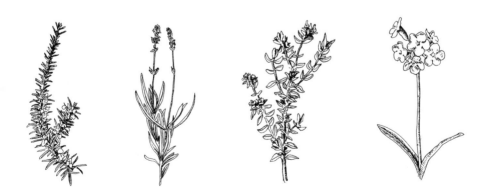

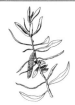

Lingle's Herbs

"The Finest Organic Herbs ... Naturally"

2055 N. Lomitas Avenue
Long Beach, CA 90815
1-800-708-0633 or 562-598-3376 Fax: 562-598-3376
E-mail: Info@linglesherbs.com   Web site: www.linglesherbs.com

Lingle's Herbs is a family owned nursery in Long Beach, California. The Lingle family have been growing herbs for over 60 years. John is also a chef.

Lingle's Herbs sells a large variety of culinary and medicinal herbs plus scented geraniums. All the herbs are organically grown without chemical pesticides or fertilizers. And because the operation is located in sunny Southern California, there is no need for the plants to be grown in greenhouses. All herbs are shipped live in 3-inch pots, so you receive herbs that have had an opportunity to develop good root systems before they come to you. They ship plants year round. But annuals, deciduous or tender perennials are shipped only from April to September.

Call for a current catalog, which includes helpful tips for growing, transplanting, best soil, watering, sunlight requirements, fertilizing and controlling insects. Plus information on how to harvest your herbs. Lingle's Herbs offers collections such as the Kitchen Collection, Gourmet Chef Collection, Lemon-Lover Collection, Hummingbird Collection, Shady Herb Collection and the Tea Makers Collection. You can visit the Lingle Herb Farm, but call first for an appointment.

The following recipes from John Lingle's cookbook, *Easy Recipes for Using Fresh Herbs* (available direct from the author), are reprinted here with his permission. If you try John's recipes, be sure to let him know how much you enjoyed them, as he will appreciate it.

ca Green Salad *with* Herb Vinaigrette so

Sometimes a meal calls for a simple green salad. I like to take some olive oil and balsamic vinegar and spice it up with fresh herbs. The combinations are endless, so experiment. The beautiful, edible blue flowers of borage make a delightful addition. ~ John Lingle

1 head of lettuce (iceberg, romaine, red leaf, etc.)
4 Tablespoons extra virgin olive oil
2 Tablespoons balsamic vinegar
½ teaspoon each: oregano, basil, tarragon, & thyme
1 clove garlic minced
½ teaspoon sugar

Wash and tear lettuce into small pieces. Combine remaining ingredients in a jar, seal tightly and shake well. Refrigerate for one hour. Portion lettuce to serving plates, pour herb dressing over lettuce and serve. Garnish each salad with a few freshly picked borage flowers. *Serves 4.*

ಌ Poached Salmon *in* Herbs ໔

This is my mother's favorite way to prepare fresh salmon. On her original recipe, we have both scratched copious notes and corrections. This recipe is the result of that, our collaboration, and is sure to become one of your family's favorites as well. ~ John Lingle

> ½ cup of water
> 2 cups of chicken stock
> ¼ cup of dry white wine
> 4 Tablespoons extra virgin olive oil
> 1 medium shallot, minced
> Pinch of salt and white pepper
> 4 fresh salmon filets, about 2 pounds
> ½ cup heavy cream
> 1 teaspoon of each, minced: dill, basil, thyme,
>   & French tarragon

In a large pan or skillet, simmer the first five ingredients for 5 minutes. Place salmon in the pan and simmer for 12 minutes, turning once halfway through. Using a slotted spoon, gently remove salmon to a covered dish and place in a warm oven. Add cream to pan, boil vigorously for 3 minutes. Reduce heat to medium, add dill, basil, thyme and French tarragon. Simmer for 5 minutes. Portion salmon to the serving plates. Spoon the sauce over the fish, and serve. Garnish each serving with a sprig of tarragon. *Serves four.*

ಌ Asparagus *with* Parsley & Blood Orange Sauce ໔

Blood oranges are a rare and exotic treat. They get their name from the bright red juice of this wonderful fruit. Available for only a short period in mid-winter, they are found at better grocery stores and farmer's markets. Here, a red sauce is made from blood orange juice, with some green Italian parsley giving a beautiful visual contrast. ~ John Lingle

> 1¼ lb. very thin asparagus
> Juice of 2 blood oranges or about ½ cup
> 1 teaspoon blood orange zest
> 1½ teaspoons cornstarch
> 1 Tablespoon water
> 1 teaspoon Italian parsley, chopped

Trim the asparagus and place on a steamer rack in a large covered pot with 1 inch of cold water. Turn heat to high and bring water to boil for 2 minutes. Turn off heat and leave covered. Meanwhile, in a small saucepan, bring blood orange juice and zest to a slow boil. Combine cornstarch and water, mix well. Add to orange juice and stir constantly for 2 minutes. Add Italian parsley, stir a few seconds. Place asparagus on serving plates, and spoon blood orange sauce over the top. Serve. Garnish each serving with a twist of blood orange rind and a sprig of Italian parsley. *Serves 4.*

❧ Pan Fried Rosemary & Garlic Potatoes ☙

This is one of my favorite ways to enjoy the aromatic taste of rosemary. The potatoes are long-cooked over medium heat to give them a delicious, crunchy coating. Blanching the potatoes allows for the use of less oil in the recipe and keeps them from sticking to the pan. One taste, and you'll never be without a hearty plant of rosemary! ~ John Lingle

16 baby red potatoes (about 1½ lb.) cut into ½ inch pieces
2 Tablespoons extra virgin olive oil
¼ teaspoon salt
4 garlic cloves, minced
1 Tablespoon rosemary, whole leaves
Pinch of black pepper

Blanch the potatoes in 1 quart of boiling water for 3 minutes, drain, run cold water over them for a few seconds, then let dry. Heat olive oil in a 12-inch skillet over medium heat. Add the potatoes and salt; stir well. Cook uncovered for 30 minutes, stirring occasionally so the potatoes brown evenly. Turn heat up to medium-high. Add garlic, rosemary and pepper. Cook 3 minutes, stirring frequently and serve. Garnish each serving with a sprig of rosemary. *Serves 4.*

❧ Oregano Garlic Bread ☙

This is one of the easiest accompaniments to any dinner. Here, the taste of fresh oregano adds a nice touch to an old stand-by. It's great to whip up when your meal needs something to balance the strong flavors of a rich entree. ~ John Lingle

4 slices sourdough bread
1 Tablespoon butter
1 Tablespoon mayonnaise
1 garlic clove, minced
2 teaspoons oregano, chopped
1 Tablespoon grated Parmesan cheese

Spread the butter, then the mayonnaise evenly over the four slices of bread. Sprinkle the garlic, oregano, and then the Parmesan over each slice. Place slices on a broiling pan, and broil for about 4 minutes, or until the Parmesan turns a light, golden brown and serve. Garnish each serving with a sprig of oregano. *Serves 4.*

❧ Herb Grilled Lamb ☙

I've served this meal to people who said they didn't like lamb, but they enjoyed this recipe. The marinade removes any gamy flavor, leaving a delicious, fresh taste. ~ John Lingle

2 lbs. small loin lamb chops
¾ cup extra-virgin olive oil
1 Tablespoon rosemary, chopped

2 Tablespoons oregano, chopped
2 Tablespoons spearmint, chopped
2 Tablespoons fresh lemon juice

Place the lamb in a shallow glass dish. Combine the remaining ingredients in a small glass bowl. Mix well. Reserve half this marinade mixture for basting. Pour marinade over lamb and coat well. Allow lamb to marinate in refrigerator for one hour, turning lamb occasionally. Grill the lamb over high heat for 12-15 minutes, turning and basting occasionally. Lamb should be well browned on both sides. Then serve. Garnish each serving of lamb with a sprig of mint. *Serves 4.*

○ℛ Citus *and* Tarragon Grilled Chicken ℬ

This is a very light and fresh entree with no added fat. It's great for a dinner party because you do much of the preparation ahead of time, freeing you to spend time with your guests. The light freshness of tarragon melds perfectly with the tangy citrus. - John Lingle

> ¾ cup fresh orange juice
> ¼ cup fresh lemon juice
> ¼ cup fresh lime juice
> 2 Tablespoons tarragon, chopped
> 4 garlic cloves, minced
> ¼ teaspoon each of salt & pepper
> 4 large boneless, skinless chicken breasts

Combine the juices, tarragon, garlic, salt and pepper in a mixing bowl. Pour the contents of the bowl into a large, heavy zip lock bag. Add the chicken breasts. Push out all the air and seal. Refrigerate for 3-4 hours, turning and rubbing occasionally. Grill chicken over medium heat for about 25 minutes, turning occasionally. Chicken should be well browned on both sides. Then serve. Garnish each serving with a sprig of tarragon and a lime wedge. *Serves 4.*

○ℛ Broiled Tomatoes *with* Marjoram ℬ

Fresh marjoram's aromatic, Mediterranean taste goes well with most vegetables. Here, the taste of broiled tomatoes is complemented by black pepper and marjoram. The Parmesan cheese browns to a beautiful crust over the top of this delightful side dish. - John Lingle

> 2 large tomatoes
> 1 Tablespoon red wine vinegar
> Pinch of salt
> 1 Tablespoon marjoram leaves, chopped
> 1 Tablespoon grated Parmesan cheese
> 2 teaspoons fresh-ground black pepper

Cut the tomatoes in half width size, place them cut side up on wax paper. Drizzle the red wine vinegar over the tomatoes. Sprinkle the salt, marjoram, Parmesan, then the pepper over the tomatoes. Gently transfer the tomatoes to an aluminum-foil-lined broiling pan. Broil under high heat until cheese becomes golden brown, about 5 minutes, and serve. Garnish each tomato with a sprig of marjoram. *Serves 4.*

Mountain Valley Growers

"The nation's largest grower of certified organic herb and perennial plants"

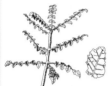

38325 Pepperweed Road
Squaw Valley, California 93675
(559) 338-2775
Fax (559) 338-0075

E-mail: customerservice@mountainvalleygrowers.com
Web site: www.mountainvalleygrowers.com

Owner V.J. Billings says that Mountain Valley Growers, located near Fresno, California, was conceived as an organic nursery in 1983 and has worked hard to maintain that quality in all that they grow. Billings also indicates that the company is the largest mail-order supplier of certified organic herbs and perennials in the nation. They ship all over the country, sending plants in spacious 3-inch pots so you get a well developed plant. They have an extensive catalog that you can order from and a very informational Web site. You can subscribe to their newsletters including E-letters. They also have a question/answer hotline. What interested me the most was their Biblical Herb Garden that includes bay laurel, Egyptian mint, lemon grass, sweet myrtle, Syrian oregano, and other plants. They also sell a wide variety of gardens such as the Butterfly Herb Garden, Edible Flower Herb Garden, English Cottage Herb Garden, Potpourri Herb Garden, Rock Herb Garden, Wreath Maker's Herb Garden and even a Kid's Herb Garden which would be a fun way to introduce children to the value of herbs. A favorite at Mountain Valley Herbs is basil. Mountain Valley Growers is a very good source for a wide variety of herbs. And their pesto recipe will make you a pesto lover.

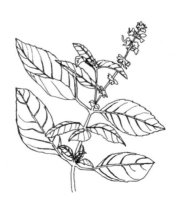

০২ Mountain Valley Pesto & Pasta ৪৩

Basil is simply a gastronomic delight. I now make about 20 to 50 batches of pesto a year and it is the most-often requested dish I prepare. It is even a hit with children, especially when prepared with one of the milder basils such as the African blue basil.
~ V.J. Billings

¾ cup olive oil
3-5 cloves garlic
3 cups fresh basil
½ cup grated Parmesan cheese
¼ cup pine nuts
3 Tablespoons grated Romano cheese

Run this all together through a food processor until smooth. This makes enough for 1 pound of pasta. To serve, the pasta should be drained, returned to the pot and the pesto added while the pasta is still hot. Mix thoroughly and serve. The pesto also makes a good spread for sourdough bread or as a gourmet coating for popcorn.

০২ Red Stew ৪৩

A favorite dish for a cold winter day, this was served many years ago by an excellent cook who included meat in his recipes. Over the years it has evolved into a vegetable stew. This makes a wonderful lunch served with fresh sourdough bread or an excellent side dish for pot roast or even hamburger. ~ V.J. Billings

5 to 6 large carrots, washed and cut into chunks
2 15-oz cans tomato sauce
2 15-oz cans stewed tomatoes
3 to 4 large potatoes, washed and cut into chunks
Salt & pepper to taste
2 large sprigs of rosemary

Cook carrots, sauce, and tomatoes over low heat for about an hour. Add potatoes and rosemary and cook over low heat until the vegetables are tender, about another hour. You can speed up the process by increasing the heat and adding both vegetables at the same time. But the rosemary should be added at the end of cooking with at least a half hour of stewing.

Fredericksburg Herb Farm

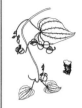

"Wishing you herbs, health and happiness"

402 Whitney, PO Drawer 927
Fredericksburg, Texas 78624
1-830-997-8615
E-mail: herbfarm@ktc.com
Web site: www.fredericksburgherbfarm.com

Original owners Bill & Sylvia Varney tell us that the farm was a dream come true. In 1985 they opened up shop on Main Street in Fredericksburg, Texas. Now the award- winning, main operation and farm, including 14 acres of gardens, is just 6 blocks from Main Street. On the farm is situated an old, but restored limestone building that was once a pioneer home for family and a cannery operation for World War Two "Victory Gardens." The Varneys have a book titled *Along the Garden Path*, a how-to book about cooking with herbs, with over 140 recipes.

At the Fredericksburg farm you can stroll through the "Classic Cross" Herb Garden, the "Star Garden," and the "Secret Garden," all filled with an amazing array and variety of herbs. Discover the "Tea Room," a café offering a tasty selection of dishes, featuring home grown herbs. On the farm, there is the "Herb Haus," a bed and breakfast inn. The "Poet's Haus" is filled with handmade candles. And there is the "Quiet Haus," a place dedicated to aromatherapy, massage, and natural skin treatment.

Be sure to order a catalog and subscribe to their informative newsletter, *Farm Family*. You will be pleased and surprised at the wide array of herb seeds, soaps, lotions, gels, shampoos, fragrances, cleansers, facials, and massage oils they offer. You can order many essential oil products for medicinal uses. For culinary use, they have vinegars, preserves, mustards, teas, honey, and a variety of taste-tempting seasonings. Candles are a specialty and you will even find gardening supplies and tools. And because this herb farm is located in Texas, they also emphasize traditional Mexican herbs and uses.

We include here a number of the recipes and uses that have been printed in their newsletter.

Bill and Sylvia Varney created quite the place with the Fredericksburg Herb Farm, which is now under new ownership. If you get out Texas way, it would be well worth the stop.

❧ Pumpkin Seed Recado ❧

This pumpkin seed paste is so delicious you will have a hard time not eating it plain. Serve it as a dip or on grilled fish, vegetables, or poultry. ~ Sylvia Varney

⅓ cup olive oil
½ cup pumpkin seeds
1 clove garlic, minced
2 Tablespoons minced white onion
¼ cup minced fresh cilantro
2 fresh epazote leaves, minced
1 teaspoon cumin seeds, toasted and then ground
1 jalapeño chile with seeds, minced
½ teaspoon kosher salt

Heat the olive oil in a small skillet over medium-high heat until hot but not smoking. Add the pumpkin seeds and cook, swirling the pan and stirring often, until the seeds are evenly toasted. They will puff and pop. Using a slotted spoon, transfer to paper towels to drain. Grind pumpkin seeds in a food processor until finely chopped. Add all the main ingredients and continue to process until well blended. *Makes ¾ cup.*

To serve, press a thick layer of paste onto foods and let sit, covered, and refrigerate an hour or more to allow the flavors to be absorbed. Pumpkin seeds are 29% protein, more than almost any other seed or nut. An early American colonist said '... for the Lord was pleased to feed his people to their good content.'

‿ Roasted Tomato *and* Garlic Dip ‿

A quick pick-me-up dip that is fun for active children and grown-ups alike. Leftovers reheat well in the microwave and make a great topping for baked potatoes or pasta.
~ Sylvia Varney

5 large cloves garlic
15 plum tomatoes, cored and halved lengthwise
1½ teaspoons olive oil
⅛ teaspoon orange oil
½ teaspoon fresh lemon juice
Pinch of cayenne
Freshly-ground pepper to taste
1½ teaspoons salt
2 Tablespoons Italian parsley, chopped
2 Tablespoons chopped basil

Preheat the oven to 450°. Lightly coat aluminum foil with vegetable spray, wrap garlic cloves and roast for 10 minutes. Leave garlic wrapped while roasting tomatoes, then peel. Lightly coat baking sheet with vegetable spray and place the tomatoes on it cut side down, roast until soft and slightly browned, about 20 minutes. Place tomatoes in a food processor with the olive oil, orange oil, garlic, lemon juice, cayenne, salt and pepper. Chop briefly. Place in serving bowl and stir in parsley and basil. Serve with tortilla chips, pita bread, crackers or raw vegetable sticks. *Yields 2 cups.*

❧ Zucchini Salad ❧

A great summer or early fall salad made better by utilizing the bounty of your garden and made special with Fredericksburg Herb Farm Mediterranean Balsamic Herb Vinegar and Extra Virgin Herb Olive Oil. ~ Sylvia Varney

2 zucchini, thinly sliced
⅓ red onion, thinly sliced
⅓ cup Fredericksburg Herb Farm Mediterranean Balsamic Herb Vinegar
3 garlic cloves, minced
2 Tablespoons chopped fresh orache
1 Tablespoon Fredericksburg Herb Farm Extra-Virgin Herb Olive Oil
1 Tablespoon drained capers
¼ teaspoon ground black pepper
2 Tablespoons grated Parmesan cheese

In a large bowl combine all ingredients. Cover and refrigerate overnight. Just before serving, drain lightly. *Serves 4.*

❧ Grandmother's Kiss Tea ❧

This tea is said to nourish the skin, act as an anti-inflammatory, a hormonal tonic, help optimize circulation, and help in liver balance. ~ Sylvia Varney

5 oz wild yam root
4 oz rosemary leaf and flowers
2 oz licorice root
2 oz lemon grass leaf

Fifteen ounces will last 30 days. Add ½ ounce of the mixture to 3½ cups of boiling water in a teapot or container with a well-fitting lid. Let stand for 15 minutes and then strain. Drink 1 cup hot or cold 3 times a day.

❧ Mini-Lube *for* Feet ❧

Here are several foot-soak solutions for your tired feet and what you have had them experiencing. ~ Sylvia Varney

Place a dozen or more small, round pebbles in a big bowl with enough room for your feet to rest comfortably. Add warm water. Add 4 drops of your favorite oil and inhale deeply while you rub the soles of your feet back and forth slowly over the pebbles. Suggested herb oils:

❧ Peppermint or lavender if you have had a long day of standing or walking.
❧ Calendula or tagetes if you have hard skin or corns.
❧ Lavender, chamomile or fennel if your feet are tired or swollen.
❧ Geranium or tea tree if you have saggy skin, blisters, or poor circulation.

We Dig Herbs

"Our mission is to educate people about herbs, gardening, growing and using their own herbs, cooking and
eating healthy, and helping people use herbs for all
aspects of their lives."

Sharee Wortman, who was the owner of We Dig Herbs, a small home-based
business in Jacksonville, Florida, sold herb plants, dried herbs, seasoning mixes,
and gourmet herbal teas; products such as bath salts, soaps, catnip treats for your
favorite feline, and an herbal doggie shampoo; and pre-packaged herb gardens
in a number of themes including Tea Gardens, Medicinal Gardens, Butterfly
Gardens, Aromatherapy Gardens, Cooking and Spice Gardens. She had a special
feature to local Jacksonville residents: herb garden installation. As of this print-
ing, we do not know whether she is still in business. But for a small home-based
business, Sharee provided a lot. We offer here, for your pleasure, Sharee's personal
favorite recipes.

‹ "We Dig Herbs" Best Gazpacho Ever! ›

> 3 cucumbers, minced
> 6 ripe red tomatoes, minced
> 1 yellow onion, minced
> ¾ green pepper, minced

Place most ingredients in food processor and puree but save back 1 cup of
combined ingredients. Then place in bowl and add to the reserved ingredients
the following:

> Juice of 1 lemon
> Dash of "Tobasco" or other favorite hot sauce
> A dash of the following:
>   salt, garlic salt, fresh ground pepper
> ½ cup tomato catsup
> 2 Tablespoons olive oil
> 2 Tablespoons balsamic vinegar

Stir well all ingredients. Refrigerate for a few hours and serve as a cold soup with
French bread. *Serves 4.*

○ Sharee's Fabulous Salsa ○

A quick recipe, heavy on the Cilantro and Jalapeño that will get your taste buds buzzing. Best served with warm tortilla chips, as a meal, or as an appetizer.
~ Sharee Wortman

5 ripe red tomatoes, chopped
1 medium yellow onion, chopped
A handful of cilantro
Salt and fresh ground pepper to taste
A dash of garlic
Jalapeño peppers, you decide the amount you can handle,
    chopped
1 fresh tomatilla, if desired

Reserve some of the chopped tomatoes and onions back. Process all other ingredients in a food processor till all are chopped well. Add and stir in reserved tomatoes and onions. Chill first for a couple of hours and then serve. *Serves 4.*

○ "We Dig Herbs" Guacamole ○

Here is a quick and simple guacamole dip utilizing two flavorful and beneficial herbs, onion and cilantro. ~ Sharee Wortman

2 packs (6-oz each) frozen avocado dip thawed
¼ cup chopped onion
¼ cup prepared chunky salsa
2 Tablespoons chopped fresh cilantro
1½ Tablespoons fresh lime juice
A couple shakes of salt

Combine all ingredients and stir well, eat and enjoy. *Serves 4.*

○ "We Dig Herbs" Salsa Verde ○

Yum! A quick recipe great with tortilla chips, warm tortilla, or smothering a steak.
~ Sharee Wortman

½ cup chopped purple or red onion
¼ cup loosely packed chopped fresh cilantro
½ teaspoon salt to taste
1 jalapeño pepper, without seeds
2 cans (11 oz) tomatillos, drained

Combine all ingredients. Blend in a food processor on the fine chop setting, let chill and serve. *Serves 4.*

Lavender Recipes
for Tea, Cookies, and Bath

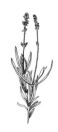
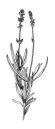

The following recipes utilize lavender as a key ingredient.

❧ Lavender Herb Tea ☙

1 teaspoon dried lavender flowers
1 teaspoon dried chamomile flowers
1 teaspoon dried green tea leaves
½ teaspoon dried yarrow flowers

This should be infused with 4 cups of boiling water. Strain and serve hot.

❧ Lavender Cookies ☙

½ cup butter plus a little extra to grease
   the cookie sheet
½ cup sugar
1 beaten egg
1 Tablespoon dry lavender flowers, finely chopped
1½ cup self-rising flour

Preheat oven to 350°. Cream the butter and sugar first. Add egg and stir. Add lavender flowers. Add flour and stir all ingredients. Drop cookies by the spoonful. Bake at 350° for about 15 minutes per batch. Garnish with bits of lavender flower petals.

❧ Lavender, Marjoram & Almond Bath ☙

And finally after a long day of life and enjoying God's Healing Herbs, *try a recipe for your exterior, an herb bath. This is a nice way to reduce stress levels and moisturize your skin too.* ‑ Sharee Wortman

2 Tablespoons of almond oil
6-10 drops of lavender oil
2-4 drops of marjoram oil

Mix the oils together, pour into warm bath while water is running, and enjoy.

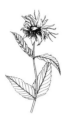

Goodwin Creek Gardens

Jim and Dottie Becker
P.O. Box 83
Williams, Oregon 97544
1-800-846-7359
www.goodwincreekgardens.com

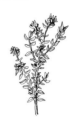

These folks are located in my neck of the woods, Southern Oregon. Jim and Dottie have been operating Goodwin Creek Farms for twenty years and can provide a wealth of information on the subject of herbs. They not only specialize in herbs, but also everlastings and fragrant plants, including a large number of native North American species. They also offer many plants that attract hummingbirds and butterflies. They ship well-rooted herbs and plants throughout the country and have a wonderful catalog with an amazing array of herbs and other plants. They also have two books available, *An Everlasting Garden* and *Scented Geraniums—Knowing, Growing and Using Pelargoniums.*

Because hummingbirds and butterflies are a passion of theirs, their catalog provides much information on what plants to grow to attract these beautiful creatures.

They have submitted the following two recipes for your pleasure.

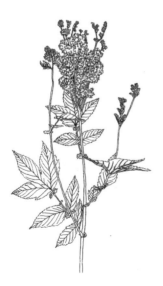

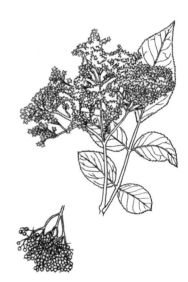

ତ Christina's Lavender Ice Cream ଓ

Here is a recipe which was created by master chef, Christina Orchid. We sampled it at her Eastsound, Washington restaurant. We are pleased that she could share this recipe with us. ~ Dottie Becker

> 2 cups heavy cream
> ½ to 1 cup dried English lavender flowers
> 1 cup sugar
> 6 whole eggs
> 1 cup of honey
> 5 cups half and half
> 1 drop real vanilla

Begin by heating a cup of the cream with the dried lavender and the sugar until it just begins to scald. Let the lavender and hot cream infuse over low heat for at least 20 minutes. Do not boil.

Meanwhile in a large bowl, combine the eggs and the honey. Whisk together until well blended.

Strain hot lavender infused cream into the egg mixture, whisking well. Press the lavender in the strainer to get all the cream and to help release even more of the lavender flavor into the bowl.

Whisk well, return to a saucepan, place over medium heat and cook for 5 minutes or until the eggs begin to thicken at 160°. Then set the custard mixture aside to cool.

Assemble all the remaining ingredients together in the bowl. Add the cool mixture, chill, then freeze in your ice cream maker according to manufacturer's directions. Serve. *Makes about 3 quarts.*

ତ Our Favorite Tea ଓ

Mix equal parts of:

> **Orange mint**
> **Lemon verbena**
> **Lemon thyme**

About 1 teaspoon dried herbs is enough per cup. It can be served hot or cold. Add a little honey to sweeten, if you desire.

The Essential Herbal Magazine

Tina Samms, Editor

142 Colonial Crest Drive

Lancaster, PA 17601

E-mail: essentialherbal@aol.com

The Essential Herbal Magazine is a hard copy publication that comes out 6 times a year and has a loyal and involved readership that contribute many articles, recipes, and herbal uses. This is a fun magazine edited by owner, Tina Samms. For many years she operated wholesale and retail herb businesses, and from this experience she decided to create *Essential Herbal.* Her publishing and gardens are located in Lancaster County, Pennsylvania. She has a vast interest is wild-crafting herbs and wild edibles, herbal soaps, medicinal and culinary herbs, and herb crafts. Tina states that, "*The Essential Herbal* is an ever-growing magazine dispersing herbal lore and uses as we allow businesses and hobbyists alike to shine by sharing their knowledge."

We thank Tina and her loyal readership for providing the following wonderful recipes.

ca The HerbMeister's Autumn Bean Soup so

This recipe is submitted by Stephen J. Lee, or as he is also known, the "HerbMeister." It utilizes some of those end-of-season herbs and vegetables you want to do something special with, plus a combination of nutritious, high fiber, protein-rich beans and legumes.

2 cups canned white beans
1 cup canned red kidney beans
1 20-oz can of chick peas
1 4-oz package frozen spinach, or fresh if available
3 cups chicken broth
2 onions chopped
1 large clove of garlic, crushed
2 Tbsp. fresh parsley, chopped, or 2 tsp. dried
2 tsp. fresh oregano, chopped, or 1 tsp. dried
Pepper to taste
¼ cup Parmesan cheese

Combine all ingredients, except cheese, and allow to cook until the onions are tender. Add the cheese and continue to heat thoroughly.

✂ The HerbMeister's Magic ✂

Here is another one from Stephen. This is a great marinade or dressing for vegetables, seafood, or chicken.

2 Tablespoons Dijon mustard
3 Tablespoons white wine vinegar
¼ teaspoon kosher salt - or to taste
⅛ teaspoon white pepper, freshly ground - or to taste
¾ cup olive oil, extra-virgin

And then choose between:

1 Tablespoon fresh dill, chopped fine and
1 Tablespoon shallot or onion, chopped fine

    or

1 Tablespoon fresh basil, chopped fine and
1 clove of garlic, minced

    or

1 Tablespoon fresh tarragon, chopped fine and
1 teaspoon capers, chopped fine

    or

1 Tablespoon fresh mint, chopped fine and
1 teaspoon lime zest, chopped fine

Whisk mustard with the vinegar. Then season the mix with kosher salt and pepper. Gradually whisk in the olive oil until the mixture thickens. Add any of the herbal combinations or, better yet, come up with your own creation and add it to vegetables, seafood or chicken. *Serves 12.*

✂ The HerbMeister's Harvard Beets ✂

If you like beets like I like beets, then you'll love this recipe of Stephen's.

8 to 10 medium sized beets, fresh or canned
2 Tbsp. butter or margarine
½ cup cider vinegar
1 Tbsp. cornstarch
2 tsp. fresh tarragon, chopped
¼ cup honey

If beets are fresh, then boil them until tender, then peel and slice. In large saucepan, mix butter or margarine, vinegar and cornstarch. Cook ingredients until thick. Add tarragon, honey, and beets and heat thoroughly. *Serves 4.*

☙ The HerbMeister's Homemade Boursin-Style Cheese Spread ❧

A final recipe from Stephen. A great spread for crackers, bagels or a stuffing for celery.

1 8-oz. package cream cheese
1 stick unsalted butter
¼ tsp. red wine vinegar
½ tsp. Worchestershire sauce
1 large clove garlic, minced
1 tsp. fresh parsley, minced
   (or ½ tsp. dried)
½ tsp. each fresh minced marjoram,
   thyme, rosemary, tarragon &
   sage (or ¼ tsp. each dried)

Soften the cream cheese and butter. Combine all ingredients. Refrigerate. Let stand for at least 24 hours for flavors to blend, then serve. *Serves 4-8.*

For more of the HerbMeister's recipes you can email him at steve@herbmeister.com.

☙ Gingerbread People Cookies ❧

I love cookies made from ginger, especially if I am going fishing on the sea, since ginger helps with the unpleasant symptoms of seasickness. Mary Ellen Wilcox, of South Ridge Treasures (Rotterdam Junction, N.Y.) probably wasn't thinking about an ocean trip when she came up with this recipe. She was making the holidays bright. She indicates that these cookies are also perfect for Christmas tree decorations.

Cream together:

½ cup shortening
½ cup sugar
½ cup molasses
Add 1 egg yolk to the mix and mix well. Save the egg white.
Sift together the following and then blend into the molasses mix and chill:

2 cups sifted flour	½ tsp. salt
1½ tsp. baking powder	½ tsp. baking soda
1½ tsp. cinnamon	1 tsp. ground cloves
1 tsp. ginger	½ tsp. nutmeg

Roll dough ¼ inch thick on lightly floured board. Cut with cutter. Place on ungreased baking sheet. Bake at 350°, 8-10 minutes. Cool and frost. Tip: If you want to use the cookies for tree hanging, make an ice-pick hole before baking.

One batch will trim a small tree adorably. One batch yields 2 dozen 5-inch cookies or 8½ dozen 2-inch cookies.

Icing: Using the remaining egg white: beat with ¼ tsp. vanilla until it holds its shape. Add 1¼ cup sifted confectioner's sugar and ⅛ tsp cream of tartar. Beat together. Make faces, bowties, little buttons, etc.

ल Oats 'n Honey Facial Scrub ॐ

Isn't it nice to know that these wonderful things the Lord has provided for us to eat, are just as good for us on the outside. This is a recipe submitted by Susanna Reppert of The Rosemary House, 120 S. Market St., Mechanicsburg, PA 17055 (717-697-5111).

In preparing this very simple recipe you can use some or all of the ingredients. Oatmeal is a must, but the rest is up to the individual. Throw handfuls of the following dried ingredients into a food processor:

Oatmeal	Lavender
Yarrow	Nettle
Irish moss	Rose petals
Elderflower	Soap powder (handmade cold process)
Almonds	

Process until all the ingredients are a coarse mealy texture. Package in jars and label. To use, moisten with water about a teaspoon of the mix in the palm of your hand. Using the fingers, vigorously scrub the skin. This is a great mix for teens with oily skin. Make it a little better by blending several drops of lavender and tea tree essential oils into the process.

ल Herb 'n Ewe Summer Switchel ॐ

From Herb' n Ewe in Thornville, Ohio

¼ cup simple sugar syrup*	¼ cup orange juice
¼ cup fresh mint leaves	¼ cup lemon juice
⅔ cup fresh lemon balm leaves	2 quarts ginger ale

Make sugar syrup, chop mint and lemon balm very fine, and add juices to hot sugar syrup. Cool. Let steep in syrup for one hour. Strain and combine with 2 quarts of ginger ale. Serve chilled. Add a sprig of lemon balm and lemon slice for garnish. Makes enough for a good-sized party.

*by volume ⅓ sugar and ⅔ water brought to boil.

⊷ Chicken Caldo ⊷

From Tina Samms, editor, Essential Herbal Magazine, *here's a great recipe utilizing chicken and lots of herbs, that will make a most favorable addition to your recipe collection.*

7 pounds chicken parts
2 onions (1 quartered, 1 chopped)
2 carrots (1 quartered, 1 diced
    into ¼-inch cubes)
1 bay leaf
2½ tsp. salt
3 cloves garlic, minced
1 tsp. ground cumin
1 tsp. dried oregano
2 Tbs. cooking oil
7 cups chicken stock

1 zucchini, cut up
1 red bell pepper, diced
1 cup canned tomatoes, drained and
    chopped
1 packet of Sazon seasoning
1½ cups fresh or frozen corn
¼ tsp. fresh ground black pepper
1 avocado
⅓ cup fresh cilantro, chopped
3 Tbs. fresh lime juice

USING LARGE POT: Add chicken and the quartered onion, carrots, bay leaf, and 2 tsp salt. Bring to a boil, then simmer 45 minutes. Cook chopped onions, garlic, cumin, and oregano in oil about 5 minutes. Add stock, diced carrots, zucchini, bell pepper, and tomatoes plus ¼ tsp. salt and seasoning. Bring to a boil, then simmer 10 min. Add corn and pepper. Just before serving, stir in avocado, cilantro, and lime juice. *Serves 8 to 12.*

⊷ Chai Tea Base ⊷

These great tea recipes are from Sue Welper of Green & Things, Vero Beach, Florida. She says some people boil the tea with the spices, then add milk and sugar. Others boil the spices with the sugar, then add and brew the tea, then add the milk. Another group simmers the spices, then adds and brews the tea, then stirs in the sugar and the milk.

4 Tbs. whole spices
4 cups water

½ cup honey, brown sugar, maple syrup, or white sugar
2 Tbs. loose black tea

Follow any of the above directions. If you wish, you can refrigerate this base up to a week, and then at serving time, heat the base, add ¼ to ½ an equal amount of heated milk, (microwave is fine). Stir well. Add a sprinkle of nutmeg. *Serves 6.*

⊷ Chai Tea ⊷

3½ ounces mixed whole chai spices (about 1 cup)
1½ ounces black tea (about 1 cup)
1½ cups honey, brown sugar, maple syrup, or white sugar

2 quarts whole milk
3-4 quarts water

Brew and strain using one of three methods discussed above. Stir in the 2 quarts whole milk. *Makes 20 servings.*

✑ Lemon-Herb Bars ✑

This great-tasting, good-for-you desert was submitted by Gayle Sathre-Zimmerman who operates The Blossom Farm in Columbia Station, Ohio. Her mail order company specializes in winter-hardy perennial and herb plants, bulk dried herbs, herbal blends, hand-crafted soaps and more. Visit them online at www.blossomfarm.com

1 18½-oz. box Pillsbury Plus Cake Mix
1 Tbs. lemon thyme
1 Tbs. lemon basil
½ cup minced coconut
1 Tbs. lemon balm
⅛ oz. softened cream cheese

⅓ cup oil
1 cup chopped nuts
⅓ cup of sugar
2 eggs, divided
2 tsp. lemon juice

Glaze ingredients:
1 cup confectioners sugar
1 tsp. each of lemon balm, thyme, & basil

2 Tbs. water
¼ tsp. lemon juice

Combine cake mix, 1 egg and ⅓ cup oil until mixture is crumbly. Reserve 1 cup mixture for topping. Pat the remaining mixture lightly into a greased 13x9x2-inch pan. Bake 15 minutes at 350°. Beat together cream cheese, sugar, juice mixture, and egg until light and smooth. Spread over partially-baked layer. Sprinkle with chopped nuts and coconut and reserved crumb mixture. Bake 15 minutes longer. Cool. Chop lemon herbs in lemon juice, let stand 10 minutes and add sugar and water. Drizzle over cooled bars. *Serves 4-8.*

✑ Cold Cucumber Mint Soup ✑

A great treat on hot summer days when it's too hot to cook. This recipe is submitted by Michele Brown of Possum Creek Herbs in Soddy Daisy, Tennessee.

Puree in blender or food processor:

10 cucumbers
2 tsp. chopped lemon balm
2 cups sour cream

2 tsp. chopped mint
Whisk in the juice of 3 lemons
2 cups yogurt

Finally, whisk in **1 quart heavy cream**. Chill at least 2 hours before serving. Makes one gallon.

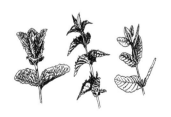

❧ Swamp Water - An Herbal Beverage ❧

Here is another one from Michele Brown of Possum Creek Herbs.
This recipe is much better than it sounds. A delightfully cool drink on a hot day!

Lots of ice
Lots of fresh cooling herbs like
    mints, pineapple sage, anise,
    hyssop, lemongrass, verbena,
    rose petals, monarda, and
    other edible flowers

Early in the morning put all ingredients in a cooler. Let the mixture steep for several hours. Will serve a whole lot of thirsty adults and kids.

❧ Cold Cantaloupe Soup *with* Yogurt Lime Cream *and* Lavender ❧

Here is another cool delight from Michele Brown of Possum Creek Herbs.

1 cantaloupe, about 3 pounds, seeded
    and peeled and then cut into large cubes
4 white or yellow peaches, peeled and diced
1 cup fresh tangerine or orange juice
½ cup fresh lime juice
1 Tbs. honey or lavender honey
1 8-oz. container plain yogurt
1½ cups sweet wine (optional)
2 Tbs. grated lime zest
1 Tbs. dried culinary "Provence" lavender buds,
    crushed and finely ground in a spice grinder

Place the cantaloupe in a blender and blend until fairly smooth. Add the peaches and blend also until fairly smooth. Add the tangerine or orange juice, lime juice, honey and 2 Tbs. of the yogurt. Blend until smooth. Pour into a large bowl and stir in the optional wine. Cover with plastic wrap and refrigerate for at least 3 hours or up to 24 hours.

In a small bowl, mix the lime zest with remaining yogurt. Cover and refrigerate until needed.

Ladle the soup into chilled bowls and garnish with a dollop of the yogurt mixture. Sprinkle with lavender. *Serves 6 - 8.*

❧ Lavender Chicken *with* Avocado Cream Sauce ❧

This one is from Susie Ditz, an Essential Herbal Magazine *contributor. She says,
'Because of the uniqueness of the ingredients, your dinner guests won't stop
talking about how good and unusual this dish is.'*

1 pound dry linguine pasta
6 Tbs. unsalted butter
1½ pounds boneless, skinless chicken breasts
Sea salt & freshly ground pepper to taste
¼ pound Cremini mushrooms, quartered
1 Tbs. minced shallot
1 Tbs. dried culinary "Provence" lavender buds,
   finely ground in a spice grinder
1 cup heavy cream
⅓ cup chicken broth
2 Tbs. cognac or brandy (optional)
2 ripe avocados, halved, pitted, and peeled
2 Tbs. fresh lemon juice
1 cup crumbled Gorgonzola or Cambozola cheese
⅓ cup unsalted pistachio nuts, toasted and chopped
2 Tbs. fresh Italian parsley leaves, chopped

Bring 3 quarts of water to boil in a large pot. Add pasta and cook 10 minutes,
or until just tender to the bite.

Drain well, return pasta to the pot and set over low heat. Add 4 tablespoons
of the butter and stir until butter melts and coats the strands to keep the pasta
from sticking.

While the pasta boils, cut each chicken breast into 6 or 7 strips. Sprinkle
with salt and pepper.

Melt the remaining 2 tablespoons butter in a large skillet over high heat
until hot but not browned. Add chicken. Cook, stirring often, 3 to 4 minutes
or until chicken is just cooked through. Remove chicken with a slotted spoon
and set aside.

Add mushrooms, shallot, and lavender to the skillet. Stir 3 minutes. In a
small bowl, mix the cream, broth and cognac or brandy (optional). Stir into the
skillet. Cook 5 minutes, or until thickened. Season with salt and pepper. Reduce
heat to medium-low, stir in the chicken and heat through.

Dice 1 avocado and stir into the skillet. Slice the other avocado into ½ inch
wedges and place in a medium bowl. Add lemon juice and toss to coat.

Transfer pasta to serving platter and top with the chicken mixture. Sprinkle
with the cheese. Garnish with pistachios and parsley. Toss avocado wedges with
lemon juice and arrange on platter.

Makes 4-6 servings.

The Author's Favorite Easy Recipes

❧ Den's All-Herb, All-Garden Summer Salad ❧

The goal with this recipe is to try to utilize everything from your home garden first without having to rely on 'store bought' items. The other goal is to try to utilize the herbs as the seasoning without having to rely upon fat-laden salad dressing.

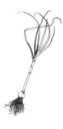

1-2 heads equivalent of various leafy lettuces such as
    Romaine, red, endive or your favorites
1-2 cups tender spinach leaves, chopped
½ cup tender, young mustard greens with stems,
    chopped
½ cup tender young sorrel leaves, chopped
1 cup of sweet basil, chopped
1 cup mixed together of the following finely chopped,
    tender fresh herbs: mint, oregano, parsley,
    summer savory, rosemary, thyme, tarragon,
    dill, sage & any other herb you may like
1 cup chopped celery
1 cup chopped cucumber (try lemon cucumbers)
1 cup chopped carrot
½ cup chopped radish
1 cup chopped red or green onion or both
1-2 cloves garlic, finely chopped
½ cup young zucchini, chopped
2-3 Italian tomatoes, chopped
1 cup, depending upon taste of a mixture of olive oil, red wine
    vinegar & herbs, made in advance

Combine all ingredients in a large salad bowl and add oil and vinegar just before you serve or serve oil and vinegar on the side. Please note, for best results, make up a mixture of olive oil, red wine vinegar combined with chopped fresh herbs of basil, oregano and thyme a couple of days before using.

Garnish with bits of nasturtium flower petals for a pretty appearance.
Serves 6-8.

You will notice that I think salads are supposed to be full of favor and to allow the herbs, oil and vinegar—rather than a prepared dressing—to provide the flavor. Your palette will come alive with this recipe, and if you are not accustomed to eating herbs, this may take a little getting used to. You get the good benefits of many different herbs, plus a lot of fiber, so you may find that this salad will help with digestion and regularity.

␣ Baked Potato *with* Thyme ␣

A delectable dish that can be served with a variety of meats, as a side dish, or as the main dish.

10 medium-size potatoes
½ cup olive oil
1 teaspoon thyme
½ teaspoon fresh-ground black pepper
& salt combined

Peel and slice the potatoes finely. Rinse in cold water and drain the slices on paper towels. Mix the olive oil, thyme and salt and pepper and add potatoes, gently mixing them so they are coated. Arrange the slices in an oven-safe casserole dish. Bake at 375° for 30-40 minutes or until potatoes are lightly browned. Serve.

␣ Italian Tomato, Red Onion, Cucumber, *and* Basil, Balsam Vinegar Salad ␣

A great salad that goes well with Italian or Mediterranean dishes or as a main dish for a great but light lunch served with garlic bread. You will find this salad very enjoyable, full of flavor and very good for you.

1-2 cloves of garlic, finely chopped
4-6 Tablespoons of balsamic vinegar
¼ cup extra virgin olive oil
6 large tomatoes
1 red onion, finely chopped
2 large cucumbers, thinly sliced
1 cup fresh basil, finely chopped
1-2 tablespoons fresh marjoram or oregano leaves
Salt and pepper or seasoning substitute to taste

Place the garlic in a small bowl and add a pinch of salt and pepper or seasoning substitute. Stir in the balsamic vinegar, then the olive oil until well mixed. Chop the tomatoes into thin slices. In a deep dish or plate sprinkle salt and pepper or seasoning substitute. Place the sliced tomatoes and cucumbers in the dish. Spread the chopped onion and basil and marjoram or oregano over the tomatoes and cucumbers. Sprinkle on the vinegar and olive oil sauce evenly. Garnish with whole leaves of basil per each serving. For best taste, let the salad chill in the refrigerator for at least one hour. *Serves 6 to 8.*

ca Mint Fruit Salad so

A great fruit salad with a unique taste because of the fresh mint leaves.

3 peaches, diced
2 oranges, peeled and diced
2 cups watermelon, cantaloupe
   & honeydew melon, diced
1 cup seedless grapes, halved
1 cup plain yogurt
2 Tablespoons finely chopped young
   peppermint, spearmint or applemint leaves

Mix all fruit together. Add plain yogurt. Blend in chopped mint. Refrigerate for 1 hour. Garnish with mint leaves and serve. *Serves 4.*

ca Dandelion & Garlic Salad so

If your yard is like mine, then come spring, come the dandelions, so before you try to eradicate them, have some for lunch. You may be pleasantly surprised how tasty this nuisance of a weed may be.

½ pound fresh young dandelion leaves
½ pound leaf lettuce of your choice
1 clove garlic, finely minced
2 Tablespoons chopped olives
Red wine vinegar & olive oil vinaigrette
1 Tablespoon finely chopped, basil,
   thyme & oregano for seasoning

Wash dandelion leaves well, utilizing only the tender ones. Combine with leaf lettuce, garlic and olives. Add vinaigrette and herb seasonings and refrigerate 1 hour before serving. *Serves 4.*

ca Spinach & Herbs so

This is a unique way to add extra flavor to cooked spinach. This recipe is best if the spinach comes fresh from your garden.

3 green onions, chopped
2 teaspoons each, rosemary, basil and
   Italian parsley, finely chopped
2 pounds of spinach, chopped
½ cup red wine vinegar & olive oil vinaigrette

Sauté first the onions and herbs in the vinaigrette until onions are tender. Add spinach, stir and cover for about 5 minutes or until leaves wilt and serve hot. *Serves 4.*

CHARTS & TABLES

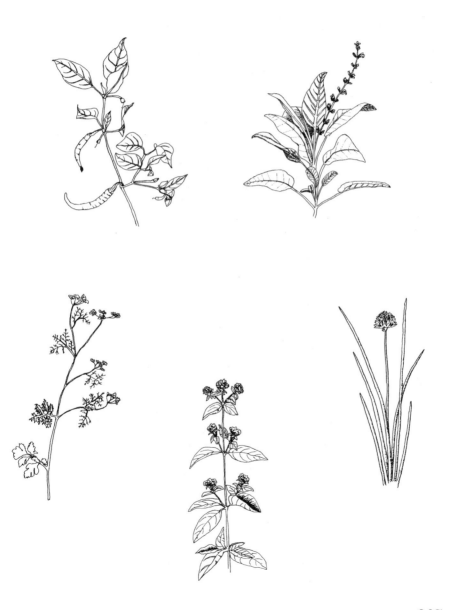

Table of Culinary Herbs

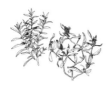 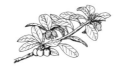 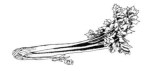

Alfalfa	Try sprouts and tender leaves in salad.
Almond	Try it in place of peanut butter.
Angelica	Use as a sweetener for tart-tasting fruits.
Anise	Add to apples, sweet breads, cookies, cakes and summer vegetables.
Basil	Any Mediterranean or Italian dishes, especially tomato, Italian squash, tomato based soups and pastas. Good also in white fish dishes. Use fresh in vegetable salads or salsas.
Balm, Lemon	Use tender leaves for salads or for herbal iced teas.
Bay Leaf	Meat dishes & stew, soups, Italian tomato based sauces.
Bergamot	The fresh young leaves in salads and teas.
Borage	Add fresh new leaves to salads. Tastes somewhat like cucumber.
Burdock Root	Add to soups, vegetable or meat dishes.
Calendula	Add flower petals to vegetable salads.
Chamomile	Sprinkle flower petals on salads or in teas.
Catnip	Fresh as a seasoning. Try a little on a sample first.
Cayenne	Spices up tuna, egg dishes, baked potatoes, etc.
Celery Seed	Use as a substitute for salt in seasoning.
Chicory	Utilize in teas. Add leaves and flowers to salad.
Chives	Potato dishes, soups, salads, fish, eggs and any vegetable dish.
Clover	Add flowers to salad for interest.
Cloves	Used in desserts, ham dishes, pickles, etc.
Cola Nuts	The ground seeds can be used as a seasoning.
Columbine	The beautiful flowers can be used to garnish a salad or other dishes.
Coriander	Add to lettuce salads, Mexican dishes. Use ground, with meat or poultry.
Dandelion	Use fresh young leaves in salad or steamed like spinach.
Dill	Use seeds and leaves sparingly because of the strong taste. Good for pickling, salads, vegetables and meats.
Elderberries	Can be used for wines, vinegars, jams and jellies.
Evening Primrose	All parts are edible and the rootstock is similar to parsnip.
Fennel	Add to salmon and other oily fish, salad dressings, breads and rolls. Sauté heads of *Florence* variety or eat like celery. Tastes like licorice.
Fenugreek	Utilize both fresh leaves and the dried seeds.
Fig	Good source of fiber, cooked in hot cereals or cookies.
Flax Seed	Add to breads and hot breakfast cereals.

Ginger Root	Cookies, candies, but also vegetables and beef.
Hawthorn	Use ground berries for teas.
Jasmine	The fresh flowers used for tea. There's nothing quite like it!
Juniper Berries	Substitute a few crushed dried berries for rosemary.
Kelp	Prepare same as green beans or use as healthy alternative to salt.
Lavender	Add flowers to baked goods, etc. See the recipe section.
Licorice Root	Try as a substitute for sugar.
Lovage	Add leaves to soups, stews, meats, tea. Use young shoots like celery.
Mallow	Try fresh, tender leaves for salads.
Marjoram/Oregano	Italian/Mediterranean dishes, poultry, soups and egg dishes.
Meadowsweet	The flowers for beverages and leaves for soups and stews.
Mint	Iced teas, fruits and salads.
Mugwort	Use like sage. Bitter flavor.
Mustard Greens	Use for salads or steam with spinach. Grind seeds for relish.
Nasturtium Petals	For salads or jellies.
Olive Oil	For anything. Try cooking popcorn with olive oil.
Oregano	Italian dishes, pizza, pasta, soups and Italian vegetables.
Parsley	Soups, salads, stews, red meat and fish.
Passionflower	Eat the fruit fresh and the juice in a beverage.
Rosemary	Meats, stews, pasta dishes and lamb.
Sage	Poultry and stuffing seasoning.
Savory	Any bean dish, soups, stews, fish and about any vegetable dish.
Spikenard	Use to make aromatic and spicy teas.
Tarragon	Traditional French cuisine, fish, eggs, salads, soups, vegetables.
Thyme	A personal favorite that I add to anything I cook.
Uva Ursi	The berries, a.k.a. bearberries, can be cooked and consumed.
Violet	Add stems, leaves, flowers to salads or baked goods. Cook greens like spinach.
Wild Oregon Grape	The berries made into a jam are said to be quite tasty.
Wintergreen	Leaves and berries for teas. Eat ripe red berries fresh from the bush.

Note:
I omitted some obvious culinary herbs such as garlic, because I'm certain you are already using them and know what to do with them.

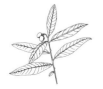 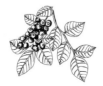

Note: Use these quick guides to pinpoint possible herb use for specific conditions, external and internal. But before using any medicinal herb make sure to consult your own doctor, pharmacist, or herb specialist.

Table of Medicinal Herbs: EXTERNAL

Arthritis	Cayenne, Fennel, Wormwood
Deodorizer	Eucalyptus
Ear	Garlic, Ginger
Eyes	Borage, Eyebright, Fennel, Meadowsweet
Facial	Almond, Aloe Vera
Gout	Angelica
Hair	Basil, Bay, Chamomile, Cinnamon, Evening Primrose, Pygeum, Ginger, Kelp, Olive, Mullein, Parsley, Rosemary, Sunflower, Yucca
Headache	Lavender
Hemorrhoids	Butcher's Broom, Chamomile, Oak
Mouth, Teeth, Throat, etc.	Clove Tree, Nutmeg, Pomegranate, Sage, Savory, Tarragon, Witch Hazel, Tea Tree, Wintergreen
Muscle & Joint Strain, Aches and Cramps	Angelica, Chamomile, Dill, Garlic, Juniper, Rue
Nose, Congestion	Mullein
Rheumatism	Angelica, Bay, Cayenne, Columbine, Coriander, Clover, Fennel, Flax, Oat, Thyme, Wormwood
Skin Conditions: Boils, Bruises, Swelling, Burns, Eczema, Fungus (Athletes Foot), Psoriasis, Abrasions, Insect Bites, Rashes, Sunburn, etc.	Alfalfa, Aloe, Angelica, Balm, Barley, Basil, Bay, Bilberry, Bergamot, Berry, Borage, Burdock, Calendula, Chamomile, Catnip/Catmint, Chicory, Clove, Cocoa, Comfry, Cucumber, Dill, Elder Berries, Eucalyptus, Elecampane, Evening Primrose, Fenugreek, Fig, Garlic, Goldenseal, Green Tea, Horehound, Hyssop, Jasmine, Kelp, Lavender, Lovage, Marshmallow, Mint, Myrrh, Nasturtium, Nutmeg, Oak, Oat, Olive, Onion, Date Palm, Parsley, Pennyroyal, Pomegranate, Red Tea, Rosemary, Solomon's Seal, Soybean, Spikenard, St. John's Wort, Sunflower, Tea Tree, Thyme, Uva Ursi, Valerian, Violet, Walnut, Wild Oregon Grape, Wild Yam, Wintergreen, Witch Hazel, Yellow Dock, Yerba Santa
Women's health	Goldenseal, Parsley, Slippery Elm, Soybean, Tea Tree

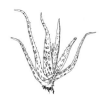 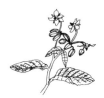 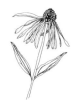 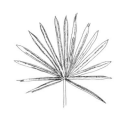

Table of Medicinal Herbs: INTERNAL

Addiction, Alcoholism	Skullcap
Allergies	Eye Bright, Grape, Red Tea, Yerba Santa
Alzheimer's	Ginkgo
Anemia	Artichoke, Chive, St. John's Wort
Anti-Bacterial & Anti-Fungal	Elecampane, Garlic
Anti-Viral	Hyssop
Arteries, Hardening	Artichoke, Grape
Arthritis	Alfalfa, Aloe, Burdock, Coriander, Grape, Meadowsweet, Wild Yam, Yucca
Asthma, Bronchitis, Respiratory	Balm, Celery, Elecampane, Myrrh, Parsley, Saw Palmetto Spikenard, Yerba Santa
Back: Spasms, Sciatia	Bergamot, Kava Kava, Meadowsweet, Passionflower, Skullcap, Yucca
Brain: Anxiety, Depression, Mood, Epilepsy, Memory, Alertness	Black or Blue Cohosh, Blessed Thistle, Borage, Chamomile, Elderberries, Ginkgo, Goldenseal, Gotu Kola, Green Tea, Kava Kava, Kelp, Mugwort, Passionflower, Skullcap, Violet
Cancer Prevention	Alfalfa, Carrot, Red Clover, Flax, Garlic, Ginkgo, Grape, Licorice, Green Tea, Red Tea
Cholesterol	Almond, Artichoke, Apple, Black Walnut, Carrot, Cayenne, Fenugreek, Garlic, Ginger, Green Tea, Oat, Olive
Circulation	Alfalfa, Angelica, Butcher's Broom, Cinnamon, Elderberries, Ginkgo, Gotu Kola, Rosemary, Yellow Dock, Yucca
Colds, Coughs & Congestion	Almond (Bitter oil of), Angelica, Anise, Bilberry, Bergamot, Berry, Black or Blue Cohosh, Black Walnut, Boneset, Catnip or Catmint, Cayenne, Chives, Echinacea, Elderberries, Elecampane, Fennel, Fenugreek, Fig, Flax, Goldenseal, Ginger, Gotu Kola, Horehound, Iceland Moss, Jasmine, Licorice, Marjoram, Mullein, Nasturtium, Onion, Date Palm, Parsley, Saw Palmetto, Slippery Elm, Spikenard, Sunflower, Thyme, Violet, Yerba Santa

Diabetes, Hypoglycemia	Licorice, Cinnamon, Fenugreek, Green Tea
Digestive Aid: Indigestion, Gas, Nausea, Diarrhea, Constipation and Cramps, etc.	Alfalfa, Aloe, Anise, Artichoke, Asparagus, Apple, Balm, Barley, Basil, Bay, Bilberry, Bergamot, Berry, Blessed Thistle, Boneset, Calendula, Carrot, Cascara Sagrada, Catnip or Catmint, Cayenne, Chamomile, Chicory, Chive, Cinnamon, Columbine, Coriander, Cranberry, Cucumber, Dandelion, Dill, Elecampane, Elderberries, Fennel, Fig, Flax, Garlic, Ginkgo, Ginseng, Goldenseal, Ginger, Grape, Iceland Moss, Jasmine, Kelp, Lavender, Lovage, Marjoram, Marshmallow, Meadowsweet, Mint, Mullein, Mustard, Myrrh, Nutmeg, Oat, Olive, Onion, Date Palm, Parsley, Pennyroyal, Pomegranate, Rosemary, Rue, Sage, Savory, Slippery Elm, St. John's Wort, Tarragon, Thyme, Violet, Walnut, Wild Yam, Wintergreen, Witch Hazel, Wormwood, Zea Mays
Diuretic	Alfalfa, Artichoke, Burdock, Celery, Cocoa, Cucumber, Dandelion, Juniper Berries, Kava Kava, Mugwort, Uva Ursi.
Dropsy	Celery
Ear: Deafness, Tinnitus	Ginkgo, Mullein
Eyes	Bilberry, Carrot, Fenugreek, Grape
Fever	Barley, Blessed Thistle, Borage, Calendula, Feverfew, Date Palm
Fingernails & Toenails	Kelp
Flu	Angelica, Echinacea
General Health & Well Being	Alfalfa, Borage, Butcher's Broom, Chamomile, Red Clover, Ehinacea, Flax, Fenugreek, Garlic, Ginkgo, Ginseng, Grape, Horehound, Kelp, Nasturtium, Oat, Saw Palmetto, Soybean, St. John's Wort, Sunflower, Yellow Dock
Headache	Angelica, Basil, Bergamot, Cayenne, Feverfew, Meadowsweet, Mint, Pennyroyal, Skullcap, St. John's Wort, Valerian, Violet, Wintergreen
Heart Health	Almond, Bergamot, Blessed Thistle, Carrot, Cucumber, Garlic, Ginseng, Ginger, Grape, Onion, Hawthorn, Olive, Skullcap, Uva Ursi
High Blood Pressure	Artichoke, Burdock, Celery, Dandelion, Flax, Ginseng, Grape, Hawthorn, Onion, Parsley, Rosemary, Wild Oregon Grape, Zea Mays
HIV-AIDS	St. John's Wort, Red Clover
Immune System	Echinacea, Green Tea, Myrrh
Insomnia	Angelica, Balm, Chamomile, Hawthorn, Kava Kava, Lavender, Mullein, Nutmeg, Passionflower, St. John's Wort, Tarragon, Valerian, Violet

Table of Medicinal Herbs: INTERNAL
- Continued -

Kidney, Bladder & Urinary Function	Asparagus, Burdock, Celery, Cranberry, Cucumber, Elecampane, Flax, Green Tea, Juniper berries, Lovage, Nettle, Oak, Tarragon, Uva Vrsi, Wintergreen, Zea Mays
Liver Function	Alfalfa, Artichoke, Blessed Thistle, Chicory, Dandelion, Date Palm, Parsley, Rosemary, Wild Oregon Grape, Wormwood, Yellow Dock
Lung Health, Respiratory	Cucumber
Mouth & Teeth	Bilberry, Berry, Burdock, Chamomile, Clove, Grape, Green Tea, Marjoram, Myrrh, Date Palm, Walnut
Muscle Strain, Aches, Cramps	Black or Blue Cohosh, Burdock, Butcher's Broom, Meadowsweet, Skullcap, Valerian, Wintergreen
Pleurisy	Borage
Prostate, Men's Health, Sexual Function	Almond, Ginseng, Gotu Kola, Pygeum, Saw Palmetto, Walnut
Rheumatism, Gout	Alfalfa, Angelica, Apple, Burdock, Celery, Coriander, Rue, Spikenard, Wild Yam
Sexual Function	Asparagus, Coriander, Ginseng, Onion
Sciatica; Backache	Rue, Spikenard
Skin Condition	Celery, Cucumber
Spleen	Chicory
Stress & Tension	Angelica, Bilberry, Celery, Chamomile, Ginkgo, Ginseng, Goldenseal, Hawthorn, Oat, Lavender, Olive, Sage, St. John's Wort, Valerian
Thyroid	Kelp
Urinary	Artichoke, Burdock, Cranberry, Cucumber
Varicose Veins	Oak
Weight, Obesity	Alfalfa, Green Tea, Kelp
Women's Health: Menstrual, PMS, Labor, etc.	Angelica, Berry, Black/Blue Cohosh, Blessed Thistle, Borage, Calendula, Celery, Cinnamon, Elecampane, Fennel, Fenugreek, Ginseng, Gotu Kola, Licorice, Marjoram, Mugwort, Nettle, Oak, Pennyroyal, Skullcap, Soybean, Thyme, Uva Ursi, Valerian, Wild Yam

Twelve Essential Herbs for Women

This list was comprised with the help of numerous women who are knowledgeable about the benefits of herbs. Before beginning any herbal regime, especially those you take internally, check with your medical practitioner. This is very important if you are already on a prescription drug.

1. ALMOND: Good for the ladies both inside and out. Almonds are good for the heart and serum cholesterol levels. For the skin, almond makes a great facial scrub because of its emollient properties.

2. ALOE VERA: One of the most soothing and healing substances you could ever rub into your skin, especially after shaving sensitive areas. Aloe vera is not only soothing, but cleansing because of its astringent qualities. You will like the look and feel of your skin after using it on a regular basis. Plus it helps with acne and healing after the harsh effects of sun or windburn.

3. ANGELICA: Angelica is a great whole body tonic with benefits to the circulation, colds and coughs, tension, headache, respiratory complaints, and menstrual pain.

4. BERRY: Blackberry and Raspberry are full of vitamin C plus lots of fiber. Berry leaves in a tea are a great digestive aid. For women, raspberry is very helpful during child-bearing years because it has a positive effect upon the uterus and milk production.

5. BLACK or BLUE COHOSH: These herbs are beneficial for respiratory conditions, muscle aches and spasms, and for a mild tranquilizing effect. The cohosh herbs are very popular for women's concerns regarding menstruation, labor and birth.

6. BLESSED THISTLE: This herb has many benefits in that it helps regulate and improve digestion, it may help with bringing down fever, plus it is considered a heart and liver tonic and brain food. For women, blessed thistle helps to regulate the menstrual cycle and stimulate mild production.

7. CUCUMBER: Because of its positive diuretic effects, eating cucumber will help your skin to glow. And applying cucumber to the skin is rejuvenating.

8. FENUGREEK: This funny-looking plant with a strange name is a real boost for all who use it. Fenugreek is a whole-body tonic especially helpful for colds, coughs and respiratory complaints. Fenugreek also helps to stabilize both cholesterol and blood sugar levels. It is said to be good for eyes (so mothers, who have eyes in the back of their heads, won't miss a thing!). Fenugreek is another herb that is helpful in many ways for women during the child-bearing and -rearing years.

9. GINGER: Make some gingersnaps or gingerbread cookies. Especially if you use whole grains and honey, there is nothing better. If you have some extra, please send me some. The spicy taste is pleasing to the taste buds and the herbal effects are calming to the stomach, especially if the kids and you experience queasiness on the road or in the boat. Ginger is also said to help with the unpleasantness of morning sickness. Ginger is good for the heart, cholesterol levels and blood pressure.

10. GOLDENSEAL: This herb has effects similar to those of ginseng as a whole body tonic that helps to maintain a good energy level. Goldenseal also helps combat stress, anxiety, nervousness and exhaustion. For women it's good externally to treat skin disorders and vaginal infections.

11. SKULLCAP: Don't let the name turn you off because this is an impressive herb with lots of vitamins and nutrients. Skullcap is a great heart tonic, it is help-ful with muscle pain, cramps, etc. It is, therefore, good for women experiencing menstrual cramps. Plus a dose of skullcap will help with stress, headaches and may help you get a good night's sleep.

12. WILD YAM: This herb is increasingly popular with women. Not for the right reasons, however. Wild yam is an herbal remedy for treating various types of pain caused by inflammation, including neuralgia. Because of its anti-inflammatory properties it is helpful during a painful menstrual cycle. Women, who seek to have a natural childbirth experience are utilizing wild yam to make the wonderful process easier.

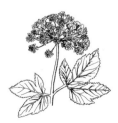 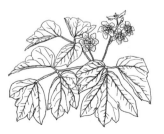

Twelve Essential Herbs for Men

In considering herbs for men, I tended to pick herbs that are recommended by experts and those that I have found that have helped me achieve a higher quality of health. I also picked herbs that will help to make up for the fact that as men, we don't always live or eat as healthily as we should. If you do these herbs, guys, your wives will be impressed. If you are on any prescribed medicine of any kind, then you need to check with your medical practitioner for possible side effects or interactions between herbs and prescription medicine.

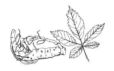 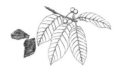

I. ALFALFA: Alfalfa is a cancer fighter. In this war we seem to be losing to cancer, regularly taking alfalfa may save your life. Alfalfa is also high in minerals and vitamins, so it makes a good overall body tonic. Plus it is a natural body deodorizer, so the ladies will think you smell better.

2. ALMOND, BLACK or BUTTERNUT WALNUT: Nuts are a great way to get proteins without having to eat quite so much red meat. Almond is also good for the heart and for keeping cholesterol levels where they should be. Butternut and walnut are beneficial to your digestive system. And we are finding that a moderate diet of nuts is beneficial for prostate health.

3. CAYENNE: Here is a way to have your salsa and other spicy treats while taking better care of yourself. Cayenne peppers are full of vitamins, help to keep the cold and flu season at bay, and will help to moderate your metabolism. And surprise of surprises, even though it is hot on your tongue and mouth, cayenne is a great digestive aid. You may find that it will curb your heartburn rather than add to it, once your system is used to it.

4. ECHINACEA: Echinacea remains a favorite herb although not all "experts" agree that it really helps with boosting the immune system. However, during the cold and flu season, I will continue to take it.

5. FLAX: In these days of fast food diets along with too-fast lifestyles, flax seed is essential with your morning breakfast. Experts believe flax seeds are a powerful cancer fighter that will help protect your whole digestive system from this terrible disease. It is also good for the urinary tract, regulating blood pressure and keeping your bones strong.

6. GARLIC: Nothing like a good steak, hamburger or hot dog, right guys?

However we continue to learn that too much red meat is not a good thing (and what the heck is in a hot dog, anyway—I'm not sure I want to know). If you will make a practice of eating garlic and onion with red meat you will find that it will help to assimilate the meat to your digestion system quicker, so it passes through faster. Plus garlic is also a cancer fighter, great for the heart and circulation and for moderating cholesterol levels.

7. GINKGO: Ginkgo is considered brain food, and in these active days where every hour counts ginkgo will help keep you alert and sharp. Ginkgo is so good that it also acts as a whole-body tonic.

8. GINSENG: Along with the ginkgo, every man should be taking ginseng, in my opinion. Ginseng acts as a whole-body tonic with many benefits and I am not sure there is any better. Once considered an aphrodisiac, we are learning that it is beneficial to the prostate and overall sexual function.

9. GREEN or RED TEA: Limit or forgo the coffee and believe that real men drink tea. I gave up coffee years ago and I have never looked back. These teas in their caffeine forms give you a gentle boost without wiring you. Plus, we know that these wonderful teas are full of antioxidants and are strong cancer fighters. And they help keep tooth decay away and enhance your breath, not detract from it the way coffee does.

10. HAWTHORN: It was hawthorn that began my interest in herbs decades ago. I was having some trouble with high blood pressure, it runs in the family. I wasn't ready to start a prescription of blood pressure medicine and this is how I discovered hawthorn. I began to take it and my blood pressure came right down. Plus, hawthorn is considered a safe herb that helps maintain heart muscle and has lots of other benefits.

11. PYGEUM: Almost all men eventually end up with prostate problems. And this is a concern because prostate cancer is a leading killer of men. First and foremost, pygeum helps to keep the prostate from enlarging or helps to shrink it when it becomes enlarged. Pygeum also has other helpful benefits.

12. SAW PALMETTO: Along with pygeum for prostate health, saw palmetto is essential and gentle as well. If you have reached your mid-thirties, a regular regimine of saw palmetto is really good for you because, like ginseng, it is a good over-all body tonic.

Other herbs that men ought to consider in their regular arsenal for good health are clover, fig, grape, olive, onion, and palm.

Twelve Essential Herbs for Children

In considering herbs for children, you will notice that I picked the safest herbs that I could consider and many of those herbs that act much more like a food. In this way children not only get the nourishment that these foods provide but the healing herbal qualities as well.

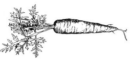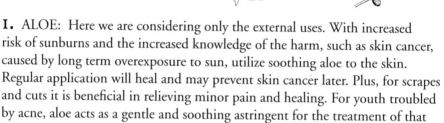

I. ALOE: Here we are considering only the external uses. With increased risk of sunburns and the increased knowledge of the harm, such as skin cancer, caused by long term overexposure to sun, utilize soothing aloe to the skin. Regular application will heal and may prevent skin cancer later. Plus, for scrapes and cuts it is beneficial in relieving minor pain and healing. For youth troubled by acne, aloe acts as a gentle and soothing astringent for the treatment of that condition.

2. APPLE: The old adage, "An apple a day keeps the doctor away" remains true today. If you encourage your child to eat an apple daily you will probably find that the child has fewer problems with digestion issues, including constipation and diarrhea. Utilizing apple juices instead of sugar and sugary drinks may also help to stave off adult type 2 diabetes. You will also find that childhood obesity and tooth decay may be less of an issue. And a lifetime of enjoying better nutrition may be a payoff.

3. BARLEY: This wonderful grain is not only full of the vitamins and nutrients a child needs, it is soothing to the digestive system, especially hulled pearl barley.

4. BLACKBERRY (also Raspberry): High in fiber and vitamin C, these wonderful fruits pack a healthy punch. I love them anyway I can get them, and as a family, we have picked bushels of berries over the years. A family outing is a great way to have some fun and gather these wonderful berries to enjoy all year long. Remember to bring the aloe for the inevitable scratches that come with picking berries.

5. BLUEBERRY (also Huckleberry): Sweet to the taste, they are perfect fresh from the garden, on top of cereal, cooked into muffins and waffles or in juice form. Blueberries help to stabilize blood sugars and help to regulate the digestive system. And they offer an added benefit: help with vision and eye strain.

214

6. CARROT: My grandson loves to pull carrots from the garden. Me too; during the season I eat about two a day. Carrots are high in carotene, which converts to vitamin A. One of the other side benefits is how carrots help with the development of proper vision.

7. CELERY: For children, eating celery on a daily basis helps keep the kidneys and bladder functioning properly. Because of the fiber and liquid, it may help with proper weight regulation. And after a stressful day at school, a few celery sticks may help to settle a nervous mood. For teenagers, eating celery could aid in keeping a clearer complexion. And for teen girls and women, celery consumption may make the menstrual cycle a little easier to bear.

8. CINNAMON: Great on toast—but go easy or spare the sugar. Cinnamon is a good overall digestive aid, and it helps with congestion during the cold season. It also helps with the metabolism of fats.

9. CRANBERRY: Cranberry is high in vitamin C, plus it helps with proper kidney and urinary function. Cranberry juice is pretty bitter, so many manufacturers load it with sugar. Look for cranberry juice sweetened with other juices like apple or grape. Dried cranberries are good for the same things you would use grape raisins for.

10. CUCUMBER: Another garden favorite for kids is cucumber. It acts as a gentle and natural diuretic, helping to clean the body of toxins and help regulate kidney and bladder function. For teen boys and girls struggling with acne, cucumber makes a great skin tonic.

11. FIG: Lots of fiber, vitamins and minerals here. Fig is also very soothing to the digestion system. If your kids like hot cereal, such as oatmeal, then fig is a great way to naturally sweeten it without having to add sugars. During the cold season, fig helps to sooth the mucous membrancs.

12. GRAPE: Like the apple a day, grapes should be considered that important. Grape is high in vitamins A, B and C, plus calcium, potassium and zinc. Grapes may also help fight off viruses, and a glass of pure grape juice goes a long way in fighting tooth decay. Plus, if kids eat grapes and such when they desire sweets, these wonderful fruits may train them naturally to stay away from white sugary items which are of no value and do harm.

Also: garlic, ginger, mint, oat, olive, onion, date, pomegranate, soybean, sunflower.

Twelve Essential Herbs for Seniors

There is no better time in your life for herbs than now. However, because often seniors are on prescription regimens it's very important to check with your medical practitioner before starting in using herbs.

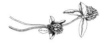

1. ALFALFA: Full of vitamins A and K, this legume is a natural deodorizer and detoxifier. It's a great all-around digestive aid and good for the kidneys and urinary tract. Because it's high in fiber and vitamin A, it has cancer prevention qualities.

2. ALOE VERA: Seniors are living longer and they are also moving southward to the lands of the sun, so sunburn and skin cancer are much greater risks. Daily applications of aloe vera will help to keep your skin healthy.

3. CHAMOMILE: Seniors seem to sleep less and less than in their younger days. Chamomile will gently help you to get a better night's sleep, possibly without having to resort to over the counter or prescription drugs. Plus, chamomile is great for the digestive system.

4. CRANBERRY: Lots of vitamin C plus a reparative for the kidneys and bladder.

5. FLAX SEED or OIL: A great cancer-fighting herb, flax is a protective for the digestive system. Flax also helps keep your bones, teeth and nails in tone.

6. GARLIC: There are so many benefits to garlic, to not use it would be foolish. Specifically, for seniors garlic is a heart tonic and cancer fighter.

7. GINKGO: Not only will ginkgo keep your brain and short-term memory functioning better, if you are experiencing hearing loss and tinnitus, this herb may help.

8. GINSENG: For both men and women, this is a great herb to keep you feeling young and active.

9. GREEN or RED TEA: Forget the coffee. Both of these teas are full of antioxidants and a flavor that can't be beat.

10. HAWTHORN BERRIES: An overall heart tonic that helps to keep the blood pressure normal and keeps the aging heart in better condition.

11. RED CLOVER: A great whole-body tonic with good results for digestive troubles. Clover is known to actually shrink cancerous tumors.

12. SAW PALMETTO (specifically for men): With the high chance of prostrate problems and prostate cancer, saw palmetto—along with pumpkin seeds, pygeum and stinging nettle—may help you avoid this deadly malady.

GLOSSARY
Helpful Words, Terms, and Descriptions

Aromatherapy: The use of scent via the herb with the design that the aroma will help to soothe, relax, give a sense of well-being and maybe even help promote healing. Utilizing herb parts and essential oils, mix in a few drops of oil or directly add herb parts to steaming hot water or into a bath, then breathe in the fumes.

Cold Extracts: This is a longer process to extract beneficial elements where you add herb parts to cold water and let stand for up to 12 hours.

Compress, Cold: The process of soaking a towel in a cool infusion, decoction or extract and then applying the compress to an external affected area.

Creams: Normally a mixture of oils or fats with herbal extracts. An example is the aloe skin relief gel that can be purchased.

Decoctions: Used specifically for herb roots, woody stems, bark, or seeds. This process calls for boiling the herb materials for up to 10 minutes, using approximately an ounce of material per 2 cups of water.

Essential Oils: Made up of the volatile oily compounds of the herb. Oils are extracted by distillation, expressing the oils, extraction, or effleurage which calls for the use of alcohol.

Fomentation: In this process, a cloth is soaked in an infusion or decoction, and then applied hot to an external affected area.

Hydrotherapy: Water treatment, usually a bath with herb decoctions or infusions added to the bath water.

Infusions: Most common process used for extracting herbal essences, as in making tea. When you put a tea bag in hot water and let it steep, or soak, for a short period of time, you have infused the herb.

Infused Oils: This is the process of using an oil, like olive oil, to make creams and ointments.

Juice: The process of pressing or squeezing juice from a watery herb.

Ointments: A blend of materials, such as petroleum jelly and powdered herb parts.

Poultice: This is for external use. It is the application of herbs with moist heat in a cloth—such as a mustard plaster—to an affected area.

Powder: Dried and ground herb parts, especially roots. Commercially-prepared capsules normally hold an herb powder.

Syrup: Sugar, honey, or similar material is cooked into a syrup, then fine herbal materials are added. An example is an herbal cough syrup. Horehound is often used in syrups.

Tinctures: For this process, you utilize 1 part herb to 3 parts alcohol, then add an equal amount of water and let stand for up two weeks before use.

BIBLIOGRAPHY

Herb Master, The Complete CD-ROM Herbal Reference Library, 1999 - 2003

The Holy Bible, King James Version

The Holy Bible, New International Version, (Zondervan Bible Publishers, 1985)

New Unger's Bible Dictionary, (Moody Press, 1982)

Nelson's Illustrated Bible Dictionary, (Thomas Nelson Publishers, 1986)

Sunset Western Garden Book, (Sunset Publishing, 1988)

Phyllis A. & James F. Balch, *Prescription for Nutritional Healing*, (Avery - Penguin Putnam, 2000)

Michael Castleman, *The Healing Herbs*, (Bantam Books, 1991)

W.E. Shewell-Cooper, *Plants, Flowers and Herbs of the Bible*, (Keats Publishing, 1977)

Jessica Houdret, *Practical Herb Garden*, (Hermes House - Anness Publishing Ltd., 1999, 2003)

John Lust, *The Herb Book*, (Bantam Books, 1974)

Earl Mindell, *Earl Mindell's Herb Bible*, (Fireside Books, Simon & Schuster, 1992)

Gaea & Shandor Weiss, *Growing and Using the Healing Herbs*, (Rodale Press, 1985)

Internet Sources. *What would we do without the internet? Much searching was done via that source for much of the incidental information found in this new edition. However, there are too many sources to list.*

INDEX

Phosphorus, 57, 117
Phlebitis, 75
Pleurisy, 28, 208
Poison Ivy/Oak, 29, 94, 119
Poison Hemlock, 32
Potassium, 11, 54, 76, 117, 215
Pot Marigold, 31
Potpourri, 14, 23, 182
Pregnant, 14, 24, 31, 38, 50, 59-60, 66, 71, 74-75, 83-84, 88, 90, 97, 104, 106, 108-9, 131, 151
Procyanidolic Oligomers, 76
Prostate, 111, 116, 120, 128, 131, 208, 212-13, 216
Prozac, 84
Psoriasis, 29, 134-35, 206
Pulmonary, 38, 81
Phytosterols, 136

R

Rashes, 19, 59, 62, 78, 92, 96 109, 155, 206, 219
Rejuvenate(ing), 53, 101, 210
Relax(ing), 39, 43, 116, 136, 217
Respiratory, 27, 48, 60, 65, 75, 79, 82, 90, 95, 98, 114, 121, 124, 130, 133, 207-8, 210
Rheumatism, 11, 16, 22, 29, 30, 37-38, 43, 48-49, 51, 64, 68, 79, 84, 94, 113, 121, 130, 136, 139, 206, 208
Riboflavin, 106, 120
Ricin, 35
Ringworm, 74, 129, 134
Rooibos, 126

S

Sachet, 139
Salicylates, 92
Salt, 38, 85, 91, 124
Salve, 22, 30-31, 49-50, 61, 113
Scabies, 60, 129
Sciatic(a), 113, 207, 209
Sedative, 36, 84, 86, 132, 171
Selenium, 117
Serotonin, 39
Sex, 75, 105, 121, 208-9, 213
Shampoo, 42, 44, 106, 112, 143, 184, 187
Shingles, 31
Song of Solomon, 13, 42, 110, 119, 121
Sores, 19-20, 29, 95, 101, 112, 120, 122, 125, 132, 134, 141
Spirulina, 85
Spleen, 40, 62, 131, 135, 188, 209
Spice(s), 42, 44, 64, 71, 100, 172, 187, 196
STDs, 74
Star of David, 119
Steroid(s), 13, 30, 136

Stings, 21, 26, 38, 99, 138
Stress, 25, 38-39, 72-74, 87, 107, 117, 189, 209, 211, 215
Sunburn, 13, 206, 210, 214, 216
Swelling, 30, 39-40, 141, 206

T

Tannins, 76, 131, 136
Tapeworm, 110
Teeth, 68, 97, 206, 208, 216
Tension, 14, 107, 133, 209-10
Thiamin, 106, 120
Throat, 20, 24, 57, 61, 64-65, 78, 80, 87, 90, 97, 101, 105, 110, 114-15, 118, 129, 133, 138, 206
Thyroid, 75, 85, 209
Tinnitus, 72, 208, 216
Tired(ness), 83, 101, 186
Tonsils, 114, 134
Toothache, 18, 39, 44, 57, 90, 100, 125, 137
Tooth Decay, 76, 128, 213-15
Toothpaste, 93
Toxic(ity), 27, 34-35, 59, 94-95, 129, 131, 139
Toxins, 29, 215
Tranquilizing, 48, 107, 122, 210

U

Ulcers, 11, 31, 39, 66, 76, 85, 91-92, 96
Urinary, 11, 18, 29, 46, 52, 60, 68, 83, 99, 111, 116, 118, 131, 137, 144, 208-9, 212, 215-16

V

Valium, 84, 132
Varicose, Vein, 30, 76, 101, 209
Vertigo, 72, 75, 114
Vineyard, 76, 166
Vomit(ing), 25, 133

W

Wart, 67, 95, 105, 129, 134
Weight, 30, 38, 54, 59, 85, 128, 144, 207, 215
Wild Licorice, Wild Sarsaparilla, 121
Wildflower, 40, 49, 63, 92, 158
Witchcraft, 7, 55
Wounds, 21, 50, 59, 61, 74, 78, 95, 97, 102, 108, 112, 121-22, 130=31, 142, 166
Wrinkles, 45, 76

Y

Yeast infection, 42, 129

Z

Zinc, 76, 117, 143, 215

About the Author

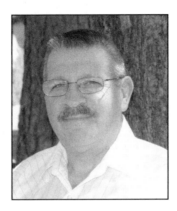

Dennis Ellingson has served as a pastor and a professional counselor. He continues to minister through a number of venues. He is a speaker and presenter on the subjects of herbs, grandparenting, and the Old West.

He is married to Kit, a professional photographer. He is the father of two grown children: Todd, who is married to Lori, and Wendy, who is married to Rob. He is also a grandfather and finds this the most rewarding of his accomplishments and experiences.

The Ellingsons reside in Southern Oregon and are the owners of the "God's Healing Herbs" research-based herb gardens. He is also known as The Herb Guy on Facebook and contributes tips, thoughts and devotions there on a regular basis.

Dennis's other titles published by Cladach are *The Godly Grandparent* (with his wife, Kit) and *God's Wild Herbs*.

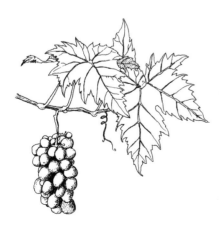

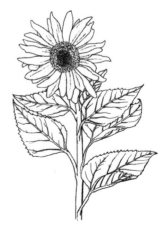

Also by Dennis Ellingson:

While enjoying God's great outdoors, learn to identify, gather, and use
121 edible and medicinal wild plants.

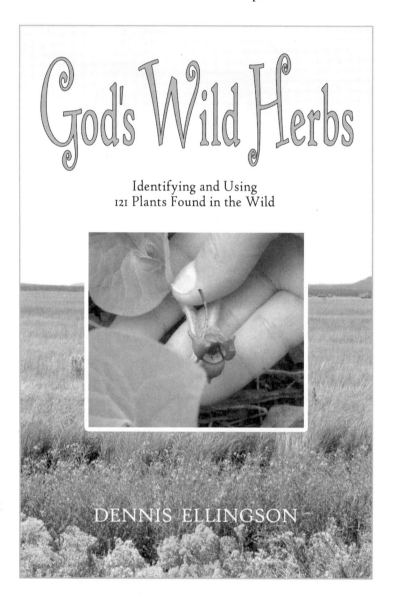

God's Wild Herbs

Identifying and Using
121 Plants Found in the Wild

DENNIS ELLINGSON

Available Fall 2010
from Cladach Publishing
and through retailers everywhere.